TEN

A Lean and Sculpted Body
in Ten Weeks

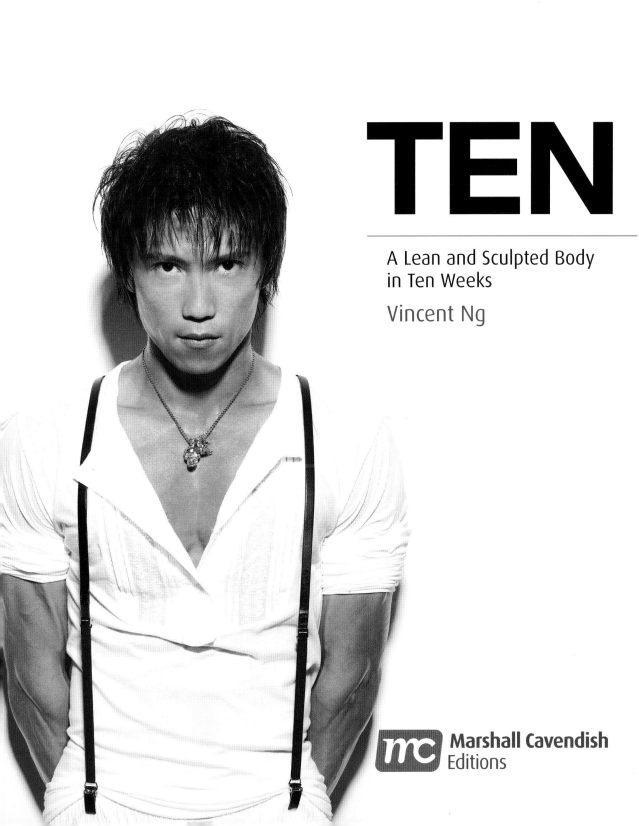

TEN

A Lean and Sculpted Body
in Ten Weeks

Vincent Ng

Marshall Cavendish
Editions

Edited by Liam Yeo
Designed by Richard Lee

Lifestyle photography by E Henry
Art direction and styling for lifestyle photography by David Gan

Exercise photography by Elements By the Box

Published by Marshall Cavendish Editions
An imprint of Marshall Cavendish International
1 New Industrial Road, Singapore 536196

Other Marshall Cavendish Offices:
Marshall Cavendish Ltd. 119 Wardour Street, London W1F OUW, UK • Marshall Cavendish Corporation. 99 White Plains Road, Tarrytown NY 10591-9001, USA • Marshall Cavendish International (Thailand) Co Ltd. 253 Asoke, 12th Flr, Sukhumvit 21 Road, Klongtoey Nua, Wattana, Bangkok 10110, Thailand • Marshall Cavendish (Malaysia) Sdn Bhd, Times Subang, Lot 46, Subang Hi-Tech Industrial Park, Batu Tiga, 40000 Shah Alam, Selangor Darul Ehsan, Malaysia

Marshall Cavendish is a trademark of Times Publishing Limited

National Library Board Singapore Cataloguing in Publication Data

Ng, Vincent,- 1975-
Ten :- a lean and sculpted body in ten weeks / Vincent Ng. – Singapore :- Marshall Cavendish Editions,- 2006.
p. cm.

ISBN-13 : 978-981-261-323-3
ISBN-10 : 981-261-323-4

1. Physical fitness for men. 2. Bodybuilding. 3. Physical fitness – Nutritional aspects. I. Title.

GV482.5
613.70449 – dc22   SLS2006029417

Printed in Singapore by Fabulous Printers Private Limited.

To the two most important persons in my life.
Papa and Mummy, I love you. Always.

Contents

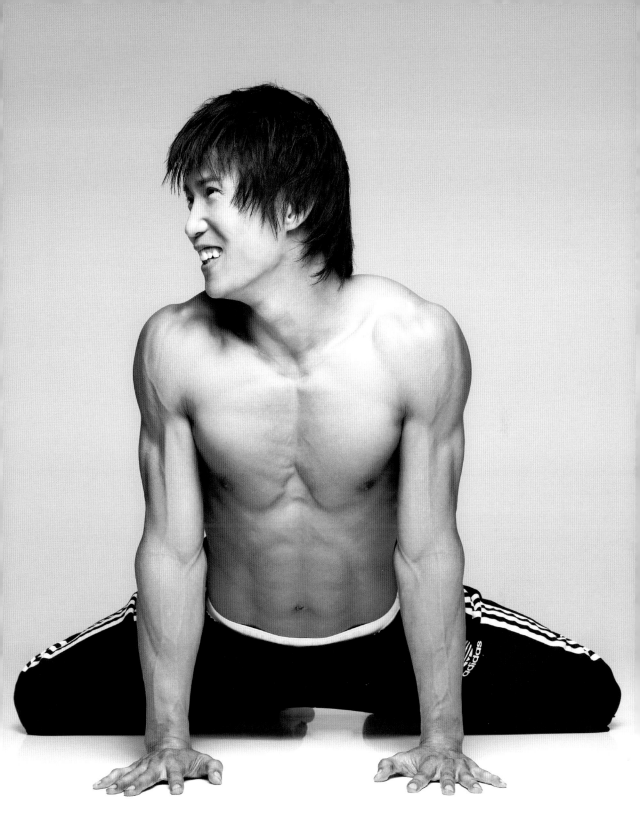

AUTHOR'S NOTE

When I was approached to write this book, I was excited but surprised. Why me? What have I got to offer? What is the book going to be about? Hundreds of questions ran through my mind.

I asked a few friends what they would want to know most about me. The response I received was unanimous. They wanted to know how I kept in shape in spite of my busy and irregular schedule. The answer to that lies in my experience as a national athlete. That encouraged me and convinced me that I did have something to say.

During my younger days, I was the best in my sport because I had the support of a team of wonderful professionals who helped me through the endless wushu and weight training, and psychological counselling. I also had the opportunity to train with the best internationally: I had spent some time at the Beijing Shichahai Sports School; my stints there really opened my eyes to what professional training was. I hope to share these experiences with my readers and help them change their lives for the better.

Aside from fitness, this book is also a recollection of my past, a snapshot of my present and a peek into my future. Of course, I had a lot of help from my friends. The journey was not smooth, but with their aid it was completed and I would like to extend my thanks to them.

There are many others I would also like to thank: the team at Marshall Cavendish for guiding me in the process of writing this book; Chee Tat, for helping me with my English, and going through so many late nights with me; James, for helping me with the exercise regime; Fahma, for devising the nutrition plans; Nelson, for giving me tips on working out; David, for making me look so good and advising me on the art direction for the book; Ros, for doing my makeup and making me look radiant; Joshua, for coordinating my clothes and accessories; Henry, for his excellent photography; James, Eric and Wee Han of adidas Singapore, for their constant support all these years; Mei and Kok Siong, for always being there for me; and Ivy for always looking out for me. Last, but not least, I would like to thank MediaCorp for believing in me all these years.

The results that readers will get from this ten-week programme will vary depending on their age, body type, gender, the effort they put in and, most importantly, their determination. Some readers may take a little longer to get results similar to mine. But what is most important is that they do not give up. The results will come with perseverance. Remember: slow and steady wins the race.

Once again, thank you for buying this book. I hope you will enjoy this fitness journey with me. Please send your comments to greenasea@yahoo.com.

The
Bare
Essentials

Know
Your
Body

Know Your Body

This is a question I am often asked:
"How did you get such a great body?"

I would like to think that I have good genes and belong to a select group of people who can eat almost anything, not do anything and still have good-looking bodies. The truth is, although my rigorous wushu training from young has given me a little of an edge in terms of muscular development and love of sport, like everyone else, I will put on fat if I do not control my diet and engage in exercise. But, fortunately for me, exercise comes naturally. Be it wushu, wakeboarding, rollerblading, bowling, volleyball, weight training or jogging, I am always game. In fact, I will feel restless if I do not exercise.

However, I recently found myself losing some muscle definition because of my eating habits—I eat anything and everything under the sun. I was also not exercising as regularly because of my work schedule. I decided that I had better make some effort to get my body to where it was while I still could. It is always easier to check yourself from time to time rather than to just let go and then suffer the arduous climb back to fitness. I decided to embark on a programme to lose excess fat and gain muscle mass. This programme involves a combination of resistance training, cardiovascular exercise and a controlled diet.

If you want to begin this programme, you need to understand a few key concepts. The first thing to understand is your body.

Understanding your body and how your body works will make the journey to fitness much easier.

Let us begin by examining the following equation:

Calories in − calories out = body fat gain or loss

Your body gets its energy from the food you consume. This energy is measured in calories. The activities you engage in cause your body to burn off these calories. If you do not burn off the excess calories you consume, they get stored as body fat. In general, 3,465 calories is approximately equivalent to 450 grams of body fat.

The trick to losing body fat is to use up more calories than you consume. You can monitor your caloric intake by taking note of the food you eat every day. But how do you know how many calories your body is burning? Your total caloric output is determined by your metabolism and activity level.

Basal metabolic rate

Everyone has a basal metabolic rate (BMR). The BMR is basically the number of calories your body would burn in a day if you never got out of bed, if you stayed awake for approximately 16 hours and if you slept for approximately 8 hours. Your body needs energy to perform essential functions such as breathing, neurological activity, digestion and cell formation. Sixty to seventy per cent of your daily caloric output is devoted to these functions.

Your individual BMR can be calculated using the Harris-Benedict equation:

For women
661 + (9.636 x weight in kg) + (175.2 x height in metres) − (4.7 x age) = BMR

For men

67 + (13.728 x weight in kg) + (508 x height in metres) −
(6.9 x age) = BMR

According to this equation, my BMR is as follows:

Vincent's BMR = 67 + (13.728 x 66) + (508 x 1.73) −
(6.9 x 31) = 67 + 906.05 + 878.8 − 213.9 = 1637.95 calories

So, I would burn 1,637.95 calories daily even without doing any physical activity.

Activity

Another factor that affects your metabolism is your activity level. This, on average, accounts for about 20 to 30 per cent of the total calories burnt every day. To determine the total number of calories your body uses every day, you will need to multiply the BMR with an activity multiplier.

Activity Multipliers

Sedentary	1.15 multiplier
Light activity (normal, everyday activities)	1.3 multiplier
Moderately active (two to three exercise sessions a week)	1.4 multiplier
Very active (four to five exercise sessions a week)	1.6 multiplier
Extremely active (six to seven exercise sessions a week)	1.8 multiplier

Taking into consideration all my daily activities, I would consider myself a very active person (I do more than 5 sessions of exercise a week). Therefore, the total number of calories my body burns daily is as follows:

1637.95 (BMR) x 1.6 (very active multiplier) = 2620.72 calories

This means that if I consume only 2,620.72 calories a day, my body weight and my body fat percentage will remain constant.

From this equation, you can surmise that your metabolic rates will increase with more exercise. For instance, if you switch from a light activity multiplier (1.3 times) to a moderately active multiplier (1.4 times), your daily caloric expenditure will go up by 7.7 per cent. That means either you can increase your caloric intake by 7.7 per cent without gaining weight or you can burn off an extra 7.7 per cent of your body fat. If you switch from light activity to very active activity, the difference is even starker: your daily caloric output will increase by 23 per cent.

Muscle mass

Another factor that affects the metabolic rate is lean muscle tissue. Muscle requires more calories than any other tissue type to survive, making it the most active tissue in our bodies. One kilogram of muscle tissue can burn between 70 and 100 calories per day compared to four to six calories for each kilogram of fat. This means that our metabolic rate will also increase when we gain muscle mass. The only way to increase muscle mass is through resistance, or weight, training.

Stimulants

Certain stimulants can boost metabolism. Studies have shown that massive amounts of caffeine throughout the day can help in increasing the metabolic rate.

A recent study in Japan compared the effects of consuming green tea, caffeine and a placebo on basal metabolic rate. Each test subject drank either green tea (containing 375 milligrams of catechins and 150 milligrams of caffeine), a beverage containing just 150 milligrams of caffeine, or a placebo (containing no catechins or caffeine). The results showed that, on a daily basis, the subjects who drank green tea burned 70 more calories than those who took the placebo and 50 more calories than the ones who consumed only caffeine.

A study by Janet Walberg Rankin, a professor of nutrition at Virginia Tech University and an expert on metabolism, showed that eating chilli peppers could also elevate the basal metabolic rate. But before you start stuffing yourself with curries, do note that a lot of spicy food in Singapore is cooked with a lot of oil and coconut milk, both of which contain a lot of fat.

Women naturally have a lower metabolic rate than men. This is because, genetically, men have more muscle mass than women. Moreover, men have only 3 per cent essential body fat (the minimum that their bodies need to function properly) compared to 12 per cent for women (primarily due to their breasts and reproductive organs).

It is always easier to check yourself from time to time rather than to just let go and then suffer the arduous climb back to fitness.

Target

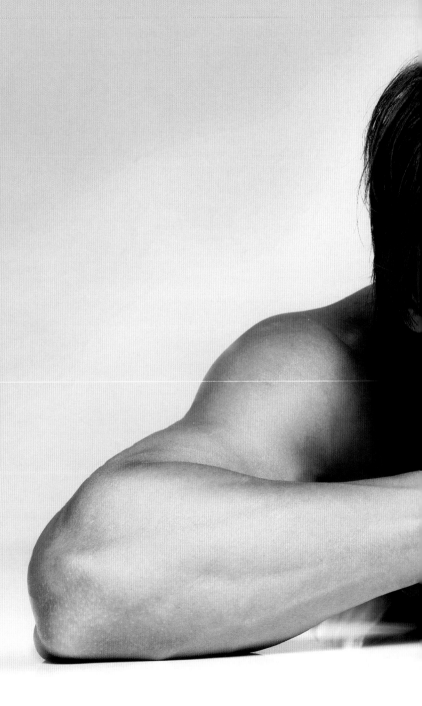

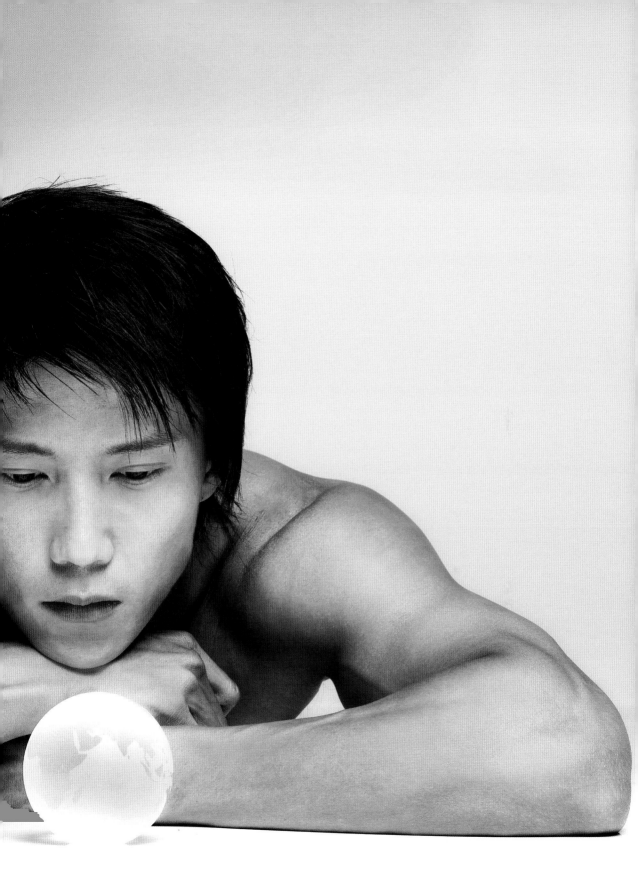

Target

Before embarking on this programme, it is important that you set your personal fitness goals so that you have specific, tangible targets to work towards. Setting your fitness goals involves defining your mission statement as well as working out achievable short-term goals. This will enable you to monitor your progress at every stage of your endeavour.

Mission statement

A mission statement is a sentence, phrase or paragraph that describes your ultimate goal. My mission statement is to become the best that I can be. However, mission statements are usually rather abstract and most are virtually unattainable. By breaking this long-term goal down into tangible short-term goals, things will seem more achievable and you will feel more motivated to train, as you know that you can reach these smaller goals. The more specific these goals are, the easier it is to monitor your progress and measure your success.

During my wushu competition days, I split my routines down into smaller sections and practised these sections over and over again until I got them perfect. This is an example of breaking down your goals. I also do not look too far ahead as this can sometimes be demoralising. I have also taught myself to take any training programme one day at a time and to motivate myself to test my absolute limits every day. When you accomplish your short-term goals regularly, you will find that attaining your long-term goal will not be too far off.

Be careful not to set unrealistic goals. Your goals should be challenging but not unachievable. Setting goals that are unrealistic can be demoralising, as you will find yourself always short of reaching your goal. On the flipside, setting goals that are too easy to achieve will not make you feel motivated enough to push yourself. When preparing for competitions, all I aimed for was to become the best that I could be. I knew that if I became the best that I could be, I could beat all the competition. I used to train 12 times a week and the training was very tough. It eventually became so bad that I developed a phobia for training. In order for me to get over this phobia, I set myself short-term goals. Short-term goals make training more progressive and bearable.

Short-term goals

My most immediate target is to have a proportionate body that is lean, flexible and healthy. Specifically, I want to reduce my body fat percentage by 5 per cent and increase my muscle mass by 3.3 kilograms in ten weeks.

How did I arrive at this objective? Currently, I weigh 66 kilograms and 12 per cent of this is body fat. This is 3 per cent below the average body fat composition of the average male.

However, when I was competing professionally, I used to have a fat percentage of just 5 per cent, and I achieved that even without a diet plan as I was undergoing more than 4 hours a day of intensive training. As I am no longer training for competition, my activity level has fallen drastically. My metabolic rate has also dropped because of my age. I really do not see the need to get back to my former fitness level and it is also not a realistic goal to achieve in ten weeks. However, I still think 7 per cent is an attainable target for me. As I lose body fat, my weight will also decrease. To prevent this weight loss from lowering my metabolic rate, I will have to put on the same proportion of lean muscle mass.

I can calculate the muscle weight that I will need to gain as follows:

Current body fat mass = 12 per cent x 66 kg = 7.92 kg
Target fat loss: 7 per cent of 66 kg = 4.62 kg
Target fat loss = 7.92 − 4.62 = 3.3 kg

So, in total, I will have to lose 3.3 kilograms of body fat and put on the same weight in muscle mass. To do so, I will have to pay attention to my diet and go through a resistance-training programme. To achieve the fat loss, the number of calories I can consume daily will have to be reduced:

Calories to lose
  3.3 x 7, 700* = 25410
Calories to lose per week
  25410 ÷ 10 = 2541
Calories to lose per day
  2541 ÷ 7 = 363
Calories needed per day to maintain current weight
  2620.72 (see page 13)
Calories to consume per day to attain target
  2620.72 − 363 = 2257.72

*1 kg of fat is equivalent to approximately 7,700 calories.

> Be careful not to set unrealistic goals. Your goals should be challenging but not unachievable.

The do's and don'ts of reaching your goals

1. Don't eat less than 1,000 calories per day.

When we eat less than 1,000 calories per day, our bodies will switch to starvation mode, which slows down our metabolism.

Our bodies are designed for survival and they will do whatever is necessary to ensure that our lives are preserved. So when you eat less, your body will slow down its metabolic rate, allowing you to last longer without food. This explains why we can last more than seven days without food.

Another critical reason why we should not allow our bodies to lapse into starvation mode is that the first thing that the body will attack when in starvation mode is lean muscle tissue as it consumes the most calories. When you lose lean muscle tissue, you will find it even more difficult to lose body fat.

2. Don't skip your meals.

Skipping meals has the same effect as eating too little. Your body will slow down its metabolic rate to preserve energy. Moreover, when you skip meals, you will also be more likely to binge on the next meal. This will make you consume more calories than you actually need.

3. Don't over-exercise.

Your muscles need time to heal and recover. By over-exercising, you do not allow enough time for your muscles to mend and grow. More crucially, the risk of injury increases when one over-exercises. Injury will prevent you from training and will ultimately ruin your plans. Allow yourself one to two days between training sessions for your body to recover.

4. Do get on the scale once every week.

I weigh myself weekly during the programme. If you miss your targets, you can adjust your plan accordingly by increasing the intensity of your workout or cutting down on your caloric intake. Do remember to weigh yourself only once a week, on the same day and at the same time and place. To monitor muscle growth, have a friend help you measure your chest, waist, hips, thighs and upper arms once a month.

5. Don't exercise to eat more.

Do not ever undertake an exercise programme simply to justify overeating. Over time, excessive eating will require you to exercise even more. Over-exercising will eventually lead to injury. Once you get injured, your exercise plan will stall and your fitness plan will be ruined.

How fat are you?

Body fat percentages are calculated by comparing the amount of fat in one's body against one's total body mass. Commonly used methods to determine body fat include:

1. Bioelectrical impedance
Scales that measure fat percentage are widely available in the market. An individual steps on a bioelectrical impedance scale and a weak electric current runs from one foot through the individual's body and out the other foot. As fat impedes the flow of electricity, the slower the current, the more fat the individual possesses. Conversely, the current travels more rapidly through muscle because muscle contains more water than fat, and water conducts electricity.

2. Skin-fold measurement
Another commonly used technique for measuring body fat is skin-fold measurement. This method is used by the Sports Medicine and Research Centre on Singapore national athletes. A technician measures the thickness of skin-fold at five to seven locations on the body using calipers. When the skin-fold measurements are properly taken, total body fat can be approximated. For the sake of accuracy, after the initial test, all subsequent examinations have to be performed by the same technician using the same pair of calipers.

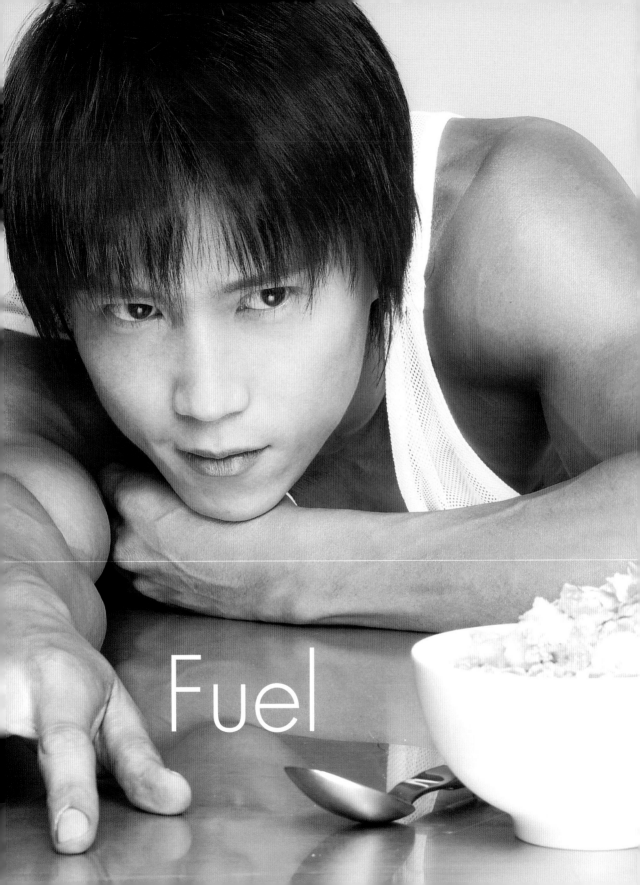

Fuel

Fuel

The first component of this ten-week programme is nutrition. We learnt earlier that whether we gain or lose body fat depends on our caloric intake and output. We concluded that one way to lose fat is to cut our caloric intake. So what types of food should we get our calories from?

No matter how many calories you need each day, it is important that they do not all come from the same source. Carbohydrates, proteins and fats are all broken down at different speeds in the body to provide a continual flow of energy. They also serve different functions in our bodies.

Daily nutrient requirements

Nutritionists from the Singapore Sports Council recommend that our diets follow a carbohydrate : protein : fat ratio of 60:20:20. Personally, when I engage in weight training, I prefer the ratio to be 55:25:20. Using my preferred ratio and the caloric target that I set, my daily caloric intake will be divided as follows:

Calories from carbohydrates =
  55% x 2257.72 = 1241.75
Calories from protein =
  25% x 2257.72 = 564.43
Calories from fats =
  20% x 2257.72 = 451.54

Following a diet low in fat is essential in helping me lose body fat. There are other benefits of having a low-fat diet, and one of them is that you can eat more. This is because every gram of fat contains more than twice the number of calories in a gram of protein or carbohydrate. Carbohydrates contain 4 calories per gram (same for protein), while fats contain 9 calories per gram.

For every gram of fat we remove from our diets, twice the amount of protein or carbohydrates can be added. This means that we can eat more, and consequently we will feel less hungry throughout the day.

While it is not advisable or practical to totally remove fats from our daily diet, the type of fats we eat makes a difference. Fats contain fatty acids, which are part of every cell in our body. However, saturated fats, or animal fats, are very unhealthy. Unsaturated fats (taken in moderation) are a healthier choice and they also contain certain essential fatty acids that our bodies require. These essential fatty acids are used to make cells and compounds in our bodies. As resistance-training exercises tend to burn calories from stored muscle carbohydrates rather than body fat, it is very important to keep fat intake low. As a rule of thumb, avoid any food that contains more than 2 grams of fat per 100 calories.

Functions of Essential Nutrients

Nutrient	Major Function	Recommended Food Sources
Proteins	Build and repair tissues. Contain amino acids, which are vital to many body structures and physiological functions.	Egg white, soy beans, white meats such as chicken, fish, turkey and lean cuts of beef and lamb.
Carbohydrates	Provide energy.	Whole (unprocessed) grains such as brown rice, pasta, cereal, pulses such as kidney beans and red beans, potatoes.
Fats	An essential part of cell membranes, they transport fat-soluble vitamins throughout the body, cushion internal organs and are a source of concentrated energy.	Plant oils such as flaxseed, peanut, soy, walnut, olive and corn oils. Fish oils.
Vitamins and minerals	Regulate body functions and make up body structures.	All whole food.
Water	Vital to health and peak performance.	Pure water, other beverages and foods with high water content (such as fruit and vegetables).

The dos and don'ts of what to eat

1. Do drink eight to 10 glasses of water every day.

About two-thirds of the human body is made up of water, so preventing dehydration is very important. Athletes who are undergoing training can lose more than 7 $\frac{1}{2}$ litres of water a day through perspiration. When I train, I make sure I replenish the water loss. When you are on a fat-loss diet, you will be even more prone to becoming dehydrated.

Even a very small shortage of water can disrupt your body's functions. If your muscles become dehydrated by only 3 per cent, you will lose 10 per cent of your contractile strength and 8 per cent of speed. Water balance is the most important variable in sporting performance and maintenance of good health.

The quality of the water you drink affects the quality of your muscles. Water from the tap has been treated with chemicals to keep it germ-free. Make sure the water you drink is pure. You could try getting one of the many water-purifying devices that are readily available on the market.

2. Do eat foods that are high in complex carbohydrates and fibre.

Carbohydrates are an essential source of energy, especially when we engage in resistance training, which requires considerable strength and stamina. When your body has depleted its store of carbohydrates, physical and mental performance is compromised. I try to make sure that 50 to 55 per cent of my daily caloric intake comes from foods that contain high-quality complex carbohydrates, such as vegetables, whole grains and fruit.

During my competition days, I did not know anything about carbo-loading. Basically, carbo-loading means to load up on carbohydrates prior to an event that you know will use up a lot of your energy. Carbo-loading is widely practised by high-level athletes in preparation for competition. I adopted this practice only when I started to weight train a few years ago. My carbohydrate intake goes up by about 70 per cent on the days that I train.

However, not all carbohydrates are created equal. A diet high in simple carbohydrates can disrupt your metabolism of fat and can also cause an increase in your body fat. I try to eat food that is high in complex carbohydrates such as whole grains and other whole foods (like potatoes) that are also low in fat and contain fibre and protein. However, be careful not to overindulge on carbohydrates even if they are of the complex kind. As carbohydrates are easily digestible, the temptation to gorge yourself on them is great.

3. Do ensure that you're getting enough protein.

Protein is "muscle food". When you undergo physical training and begin to develop more muscle tissue, your body will require more protein to repair, maintain and grow your muscle cells.

In addition to making muscle tissue, proteins have other important functions. Proteins are made up of amino acids. Amino acids also form enzymes that are needed to make your body run correctly. They are also used to make neuro-chemicals that are used in your brain and nervous system. Since it is our nervous system that controls our muscles, it makes sense to keep it well nourished.

4. Do stick to a diet low in saturated fat and cholesterol.

There are good fats and bad fats. Saturated fats are bad fats and should be eliminated from your diet. Almost all saturated fats, such as animal fat, are solid at room temperature. Most foods high in saturated fats are low in essential fatty acids and high in cholesterol.

Food that is higher in unsaturated and polyunsaturated fats can lower cholesterol levels and reduce the risk of heart disease. These fats, found in plant and fish oils, tend to be high in essential fatty acids, which have many beneficial effects on the body.

However, food processing can change unsaturated fats into semi-saturated ones. Although most saturated fats are solid at room temperature, this does not mean that all oils that are liquid at room temperature are unsaturated. Coconut oil, for example, is liquid but is primarily composed of saturated fats.

5. Don't consume processed foods.

When sugar or flour is processed or refined, much of the fibre and nutrients in them is also removed in the process. Fibre regulates digestion; it slows down digestion to a healthy rate. When your diet is high in refined and processed food, it is lower in fibre and essential nutrients.

Besides being a source of "empty calories", some processed foods may actually be harmful to your health. It has been suggested that refined sugar, for example, surges through the body too rapidly, causing the release of chemicals called free radicals, which have been associated with aging and heart disease. This is why complex carbohydrates are preferable. They do not rush through your system and overwhelm it.

6. Do lower your salt intake.

Salt is an essential mineral; if we do not get enough of it, our health and athletic performance will be affected. However, if we consume too much of it, our health will also be damaged. Besides causing serious health problems such as high blood pressure, taking too much salt will also upset our bodies' water balance, which can slow us down. As most of our diets are already too high in salt, we need to cut back on seasoning our food and on our consumption of packaged (canned or preserved) food.

7. Don't indulge in fast food.

Fast food often contains too much sugar, saturated fats, cholesterol and salt. Most fast-food products have very little to offer in terms of complex carbohydrates, protein, fibre, essential fatty acids, vitamins and minerals. Need I say more?

When to eat: the secret to losing fat and building muscle

Instead of taking three meals a day, we should spread out our calorie intake into five or six lighter meals. Our bodies can only use a limited number of calories every hour. If we eat too much in one meal, the excess calories will end up getting converted to fats, which in turn, get stored as body fat. If we spread out our calorie intake, we ensure that the calories that we consume are used more efficiently.

However, remember that this is not the same as overeating. The number of calories that you require does not change; the only difference is that you divide up all the food you need each day into five parts instead of three.

By eating (not overeating) more regularly, we force our bodies to constantly burn calories while preventing them from switching into starvation mode. This will raise and stabilise our metabolic rate, ensuring that all the calories that we consume are used up and not stored as body fat.

The dos and don'ts of when to eat

1. Do have regular meals.

By skipping meals, we starve our bodies and our bodies will start to attack our lean muscle mass. Our lean muscle mass is the biggest spender of calories and, if no calories are consumed, our bodies will attack (digest) our lean muscle mass first in an attempt to reduce the calories we burn. This will not only lower our metabolic rate but also put all our time and effort in building lean muscle tissue at the gym to waste!

2. Do stop snacking at least 3 hours before bedtime.

If you have a supper habit, now is the time to quit it. If we eat just before turning in for the night, our bodies are likely to store the calories from supper as unwanted fat. However, going to bed hungry can also trigger off the same starvation mode that skipping breakfast initiates, encouraging our bodies to store any excess calories as fat. If you really have to eat before bedtime, then turn to steamed vegetables or fruit.

My colleagues often invite me to join them for supper after late night film shoots. I used to oblige until I realised that my weight was being adversely affected by those late night meals. Now I will still join them for supper, but instead of eating, I normally just order a low-calorie drink. If I do work late into the night, I will eat while I am filming (most likely 3 hours before I go to bed) rather than after work. This will ensure that I do not go to bed hungry.

Eating before, during and after exercise

I try to consume a low-fat meal that is high in carbohydrates and protein about 2 to 3 hours before my training sessions. This ensures that I have enough energy to last the whole workout.

Although we tend to perspire very little during resistance training, a lot of water actually goes into our muscle cells when we lift weights. Failing to replenish this water loss will result in dehydration. Besides water, sports drinks can be useful in making up for the minerals and salts lost during the workout.

About half an hour to an hour after a workout, have a meal that is high in complex carbohydrates to help your body construct muscle tissues more efficiently.

The meal plan

The sample meal plans on pages 32 to 37 are designed to adhere to a carbohydrate : protein : fat ratio of 55:25:20. Depending on your total caloric output and the target you set, choose the nutritional plan that suits you best.

As with all diets, discipline is key. On the other hand, be realistic. Do not attempt to follow a diet that you know you cannot stick to. You will yield much better results with a diet that you can follow throughout the ten weeks rather than with one you will end after only one week.

From time to time, you may wish to reward yourself (do this sparingly). Use the local food calorie counter on page 38 to calculate how many calories you can consume for the rest of the day after you indulge.

Which makes more sense?

Having small regular meals will also stop us from binging at mealtimes. You may be familiar with this scenario: you skip breakfast because you wake up late and have to rush to work. You run on empty for the most part of the morning and your body soon switches to starvation mode. By lunchtime, you are totally famished. Before you know it, you have overeaten. The calories that you consume far exceed what your body needs. The excess ends up being converted to body fat. For the rest of the afternoon, you cannot find time to grab a bite and your body switches to starvation mode again. By the time dinner is served, you are so ravenous that you binge, and the vicious circle begins again.

This is the alternative: You make sure you have breakfast every day. Your body is constantly working in peak condition to burn off the calories. By around 10 am, the calories would have been burned off. You eat a small snack (which takes you less than 5 minutes to finish) and that provides the body with the calories necessary to operate optimally; no calories are converted into fat. By lunchtime, you do not feel that hungry and you have a light lunch; you do not overeat. Just as in the morning, you have a small snack in the afternoon. When it is time for dinner, you are not overly hungry and you have a light dinner. All the calories that you consumed on this day have been effectively used up without being stored as body fat.

No matter how many calories you need each day, it is important that they do not all come from the same source.

Meal Plan—1800 kcals

	Monday	Tuesday	Wednesday
Breakfast	2 chee cheong fun rolls (minimal oil) 1 cup of tea with milk	A slice of thinly buttered raisin toast 2 soft-boiled eggs 1 cup of Milo with milk	2 slices of toast with low-fat cheese 1 cup of soy bean milk
Lunch	1 bowl of yong tau foo beehoon soup 2 slices of fruit 1 cup of water	A plate of rice with stir-fried chicken (skin removed) and green, leafy vegetables 1 cup of fruit juice	1 bowl of sliced fish soup (extra serving of fish) with yam rice 2 slices of fruit 1 cup of water
Afternoon tea	2 slices of fruit or 1 tuna sandwich (2 slices of bread and tuna in brine) A cup of coffee or tea	2 slices of fruit or 1 red bean bun 1 cup of coffee or tea	2 slices of fruit or 1 sugar bun 1 cup of coffee or tea
Dinner	1 plate of rice with ¼ dry roasted chicken and green leafy vegetables 1 glass of water	1 bowl of handmade noodles 1 bowl of ice jelly	1 plate of beef hor fun and vegetables 1 cup of green tea

Thursday	Friday	Saturday	Sunday
1 bowl of cereal with 200ml of low-fat milk 1 banana 1 cup of tea with milk	2 slices of toast thinly spread with Nutella 2 soft-boiled eggs 1 cup of soy bean milk	2 pancakes lightly drizzled with maple syrup 1 cup Milo with milk	1 bowl of cereal with 200ml low-fat milk 1 cup of tea with milk
1 plate of rice with seafood stir-fry in tomato sauce 1 cup of fruit juice	1 bowl of beef ball or sliced beef soup with rice or noodles 2 slices of fruit 1 cup of water	1 plate of duck (skin removed) rice with vegetables and 1 piece of firm bean curd 1 cup of fruit juice	1 sandwich with low-fat filling 1 cup of a sweetened drink
2 slices of fruit or 1 chocolate bun 1 cup of coffee or tea	2 slices of fruit or 2 slices of bread with low-fat cheese 1 cup of coffee or tea	2 slices of fruit or 1 raisin bun 1 cup of coffee or tea	2 slices of fruit 1 cup of coffee or tea
1 bowl of fish ball noodles with vegetables 1 cup of water	1 plate of fried beehoon with sliced chicken and mixed vegetables 1 cup of water	1 plate of rice with grilled fish and green vegetables 1 cup of a sweetened drink	1 plate of seafood pasta in a tomato sauce 1 cup of water

Meal Plan—2300 kcals

	Monday	Tuesday	Wednesday
Breakfast	4 slices of bread with egg omelette A cup of Milo with milk	1 bowl of cereal with sliced bananas and milk 2 slices of raisin bread A cup of coffee or tea	3 pancakes lightly drizzled with maple syrup 2 soft-boiled eggs A cup of Milo with milk
Snack	2 slices of raisin bread	1 cereal bar	1 steamed bun
Lunch	1 bowl of duck (skin removed) noodles (extra serving of meat) 1 slice of watermelon 1 bowl of ice jelly	1 bowl of handmade noodle soup 1 slice of papaya 1 bowl of sweet green bean soup	1 plate of seafood pasta in tomato sauce 2 buns ½ mango
Snack	1 small tub of low-fat yoghurt	1 small packet of low-fat milk	1 small packet of low-fat yogurt drink
Dinner	1 plate of rice 1 bowl of sliced fish soup (extra serving of fish) and vegetables 1 glass of fruit juice	1 plate of rice with chicken (skin removed) teriyaki and stir-fried chye sim 1 glass soy bean drink	1 plate of rice with lean beef teppanyaki and stir-fried kailan 1 can of herbal tea

Thursday	Friday	Saturday	Sunday
1 bowl of century egg porridge 1 steamed bun 1 glass of low-fat milk	4 slices of bread with ham, lettuce and tomato 1 cup of soy bean milk	1 bowl of oat porridge with milk 2 slices of banana bread A cup of coffee or tea	3 slices of French toast 2 soft-boiled eggs A cup of Milo with milk
1 slice of pandan chiffon cake	1 cheese bun	1 cereal bar	1 can of iced Milo
1 bowl of yong tauhu beehoon soup 1 bowl of almond jelly 1 slice of honeydew melon	1 plate of rice with stir-fried lean beef and green, leafy vegetables 2 kiwifruits	1 plate of rice with lemon chicken and stir-fried broccoli 2 slices of pineapple	1 bowl of mee soto 2 hard-boiled eggs 1 bowl of sweet red bean soup
1 packet of Milo	1 packet of soy milk	1 tub of low-fat yoghurt	1 packet of low-fat milk
1 plate of rice with grilled fish fillet and stir-fried cabbage 1 can of green tea	1 plate of rice with curried chicken (skin removed), potato and vegetables ½ mango 1 can of herbal tea	1 plate of pasta with fish in tomato sauce 1 bowl of green salad with a low-fat dressing 1 cup of coffee or tea	1 plate of rice with black pepper beef and stir-fried spinach 1 can of green tea

Meal Plan—2600 kcals

	Monday	Tuesday	Wednesday
Breakfast	4 slices of bread with egg omelette 1 cup of Milo with milk	1 bowl of cereal with sliced bananas and milk 2 slices of raisin bread 1 cup of coffee or tea	3 pancakes with maple syrup 2 soft-boiled eggs 1 cup of Milo with milk
Snack	2 slices of raisin bread 1 tub of low-fat yoghurt	1 cereal bar 1 packet of low-fat milk	1 steamed bun 1 packet of a low-fat yogurt drink
Lunch	1 plate of duck (skin removed) noodles (extra portion of meat) 1 slice of watermelon 1 bowl of ice jelly	1 bowl of ban mian soup 1 slice of papaya 1 bowl of sweet green bean soup	1 plate of seafood pasta in tomato sauce 2 buns ½ mango
Snack	2 low-fat cheese sandwiches 1 cup of coffee or tea	2 smoked salmon sandwiches 1 cup of coffee or tea	2 egg sandwiches 1 cup of coffee or tea
Dinner	1 plate of rice 1 bowl of sliced fish soup (extra portion of fish) with vegetables 1 glass of fruit juice	1 plate of rice with chicken (skin removed) teriyaki and stir-fried chye sim 1 glass of soy bean drink	1 plate of rice with lean beef teppanyaki and stir-fried kailan 1 can of herbal tea

Thursday	Friday	Saturday	Sunday
1 bowl of century egg porridge 1 steamed bun 1 glass of low-fat milk	4 slices of bread with ham, lettuce and tomato 1 cup of soy bean milk	1 bowl of oat porridge with milk 2 slices of banana bread 1 cup of coffee or tea	3 slices of French toast 2 soft-boiled eggs 1 cup of Milo with milk
1 slice of pandan chiffon cake 1 packet of Milo	1 cheese bun 1 packet of soy milk	1 cereal bar 1 tub of low-fat yoghurt	6 wheat biscuits 1 can of iced Milo
1 bowl of yong tauhu beehoon soup 1 bowl of almond jelly 1 slice of honeydew melon	1 plate of rice with stir-fried lean beef and green vegetables 2 kiwifruit	1 plate of rice with lemon chicken and stir-fried broccoli 2 slices of pineapple	1 bowl of mee soto with 2 hard-boiled eggs 1 bowl of sweet red bean soup 1 orange
2 roast beef (lean) sandwiches 1 cup of coffee or tea	2 tuna (tuna in brine) sandwiches 1 cup of coffee or tea	2 egg sandwiches 1 cup of coffee or tea	2 turkey ham sandwiches A cup of coffee or tea
1 plate of rice with grilled fish fillet and stir-fried cabbage 1 can of green tea	1 plate of rice with curried chicken (skin removed), potato and vegetables ½ mango 1 can of herbal tea	1 plate of pasta with fish in tomato sauce 1 bowl of a green salad with low-fat dressing 1 cup of coffee or tea	1 plate of rice with black pepper beef and stir-fried spinach 1 can of green tea

Local Food Calorie Counter

Dish	Serving size	Calories
Ban mian soup	1 bowl	475
Beef hor fun	1 plate	697
Chicken rice	1 plate	620
Deep-fried spring chicken	½ chicken	530
Duck rice	1 plate	672
Fish ball noodles (dry)	1 bowl	550
Fish ball noodles (soup)	1 bowl	370
Fish beehoon soup	1 bowl	350
Fried carrot cake	1 plate	470
Fried kuay teow	1 plate	741
Fried oyster omelette	1 plate	645
Fried rice	1 plate	907
Hokkien mee	1 plate	522
Hong Kong fried noodles	1 plate	694
Laksa	1 bowl	670
Mee goreng	1 plate	500
Nasi lemak	1 plate	494
Pork chop	1 plate	730
Roti prata with curry	1 slice	130
Egg roti prata with curry	1 slice	318
Wonton noodles (dry)	1 bowl	405
Wonton noodles (soup)	1 plate	396

"For every gram of fat we remove from our diets, twice the amount of protein or carbohydrates can be added."

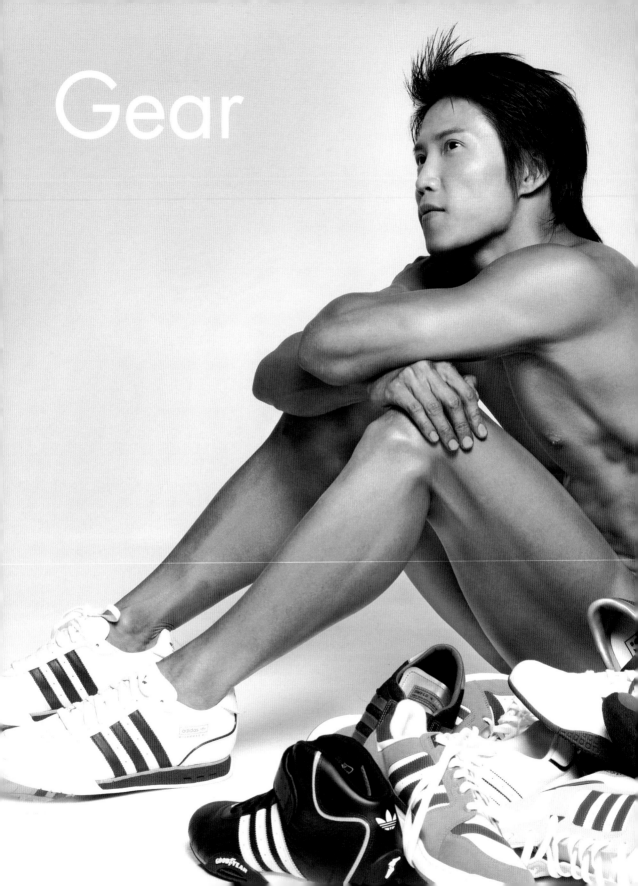

Gear

Gear

We have set our goals, understood our bodies and learnt about nutrition. We are ready to begin the programme. The first thing we need to do is to get the appropriate gear.

Shoes

Good posture starts at the feet so it is important to take good care of them. If you have not been exercising for a long time, it is advisable to buy a new pair of shoes. The old pair of trainers from the closet might look new and unused but their support structure could already be weakened. A good pair of shoes will provide the necessary support to the arch and heel of your feet. When engaged in a fitness programme, be prepared to change your exercise shoes every three to four months.

Remember to use these shoes only for your gym workouts. Different sports put stress on different parts of your feet, so sports shoes are designed with different support structures.

This is why we do not use our basketball shoes for running or our tennis shoes for football. Using shoes that are not meant for a sport will eventually lead to injury.

Apparel

Wear lightweight clothing that will allow your skin to "breathe". This will enable perspiration to evaporate, helping to lower your body temperature, and prevent overheating. You can exercise longer when your body is cooler.

Heart rate monitor

A heart rate monitor will give you valuable information on how your body is responding to exercise. It is useful to monitor your heart rate throughout your cardiovascular training sessions. You can use this information to adjust the exercise intensity to maximise the effects of the workout.

"If you have not been exercising for a long time, it is advisable to buy a new pair of shoes. The old pair of trainers from the closet might look new and unused but their support structure could already be weakened.

Some heart rate monitors can even calculate the total number of calories burnt after each exercise. This is very useful for customising your diet.

Gyms and instructors

A well-equipped gym will have a combination of free weights and machines. With a wide range of equipment, club members will be able to perform a range of exercises that will target every part of their bodies, thereby minimising the risk of injury. One of the main causes of injury at the gym is over-training a particular muscle group while neglecting other muscle groups.

Joining a gym can cost between $30 a month, for a small public gym, and $200 a month, for a private one. Private gyms will give you access to top of the range equipment without the stress of having to queue for them. However, if you do not mind the wait, public gyms do offer an adequate range of exercise equipment in the residential heartlands.

Another good way to prevent training injuries is to work with a certified personal trainer. Fitness instructors will be able to correct your technique, and can be a great source of motivation and encouragement during your training sessions.

Personal trainers generally charge between $50 and $120 per session, depending on their credentials and experience. If you choose to engage a trainer, choose one who is certified by sports schools and institutions such as the American College of Sports Medicine and the Asian Academy for Sports and Fitness Professionals. They should also be able to give CPR and first aid.

Exercise equipment

We may not always be able to afford the time to go to a gym. With the following exercise equipment, we can perform a wide range of exercises at home or even in the hotel room when we are travelling abroad.

1. Exercise tubing

Exercise tubing, which comes in different colour-coded tensions, is predominantly used for the upper body. For the lower body, exercise rings, placed around the legs, provide great resistance for working the calves and the hamstrings.

2. Exercise ball

This is a large inflatable ball that comes in various sizes and can be used in a variety of exercises. It helps you focus the exercise on the core of your body, including the abdominals and the lower back. It is also great for creating instability in your exercises, which is useful when you are trying to incorporate progression into your routine.

3. Free weights

Dumbbells can be used to train various parts of the body. Start with a pair of three-, five-, eight-, ten-, twelve- and fifteen-pound weights. Alternatively, there are dumbbells that allow you to change the weight on the bar. However, I find it very cumbersome having to keep changing the weights for each exercise I do.

4. Weighing machine

An electronic weighing machine is essential. I like those that include functions that measure body fat and water composition. They help me monitor my body fat and lean muscle weight.

"Private gyms will give you access to top of the range equipment without the stress of having to queue for them. However, if you do not mind the wait, public gyms do offer an adequate range of exercise equipment in the residential heartlands."

The
Regime

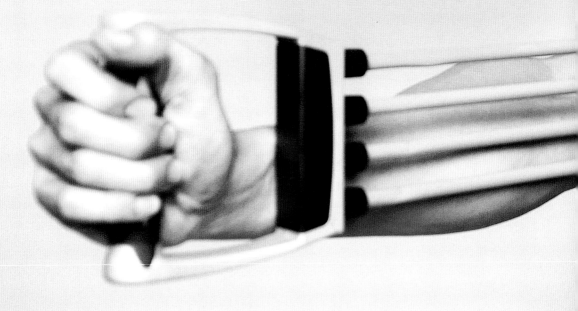

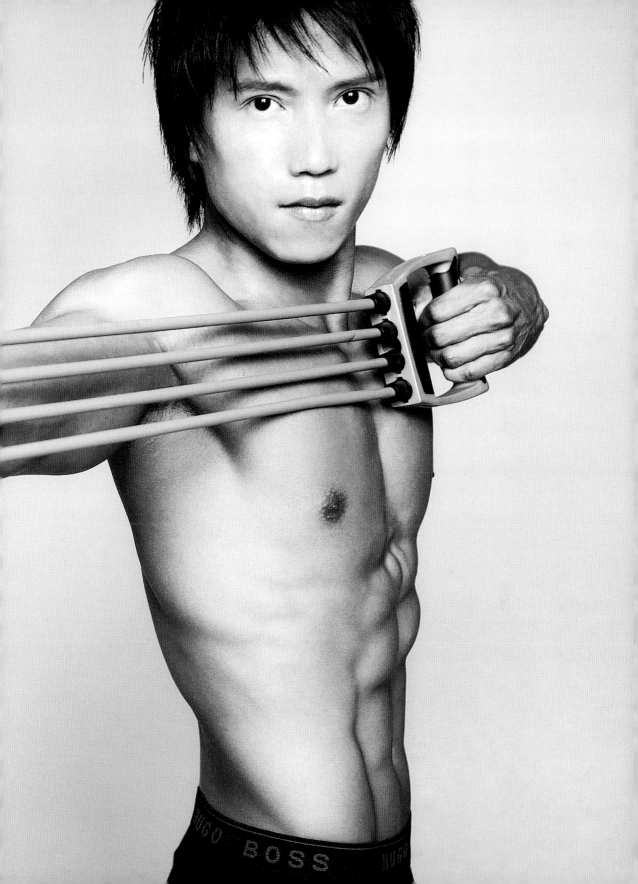

Although this ten-week programme consists of both cardiovascular exercises and resistance training, it focuses primarily on strength and resistance training.

I am going to allocate 25 per cent of my workout time to cardiovascular exercise and 75 per cent to strength and resistance training. As it is commonly held that the key to losing body fat is cardiovascular exercise, you may be wondering about this programme's focus on strength and resistance training.

A friend once made a very interesting observation that I think may go some way in explaining why resistance training is key to losing fat. Walk into the cardiovascular exercise stations of any health club or gym. What do you see there? Dozens and dozens of people on treadmills, Stairmasters, bikes and other assorted cardiovascular exercise equipment. Notice that, although many of these people are on these machines for hours on end each week, the majority of them are overweight. Next, take a look at the people working out with strength and resistance equipment. The people here are also training very hard. However, notice that the majority of them are in far better shape than the people

at the cardiovascular section. So, in which section do you want to spend more time?

Think of it this way: Cardiovascular exercise trains the most important muscle in our body— our heart. But it predominantly trains only that one muscle. What about the rest of our muscles? Devoting 25 per cent of your regime to one muscle is sufficient to work that muscle. Giving 75 per cent of your exercise effort to the rest of your body is thus a logical approach.

Through strength and resistance training, we build lean muscle mass, which is the body tissue that consumes the most calories. This translates to a higher metabolism all day long. (I will discuss the benefits of strength and resistance training in more detail in the next chapter, Build.)

Nonetheless, cardiovascular exercise is necessary in our programme as it benefits our bodies. The American Medical Association states that 20 minutes of cardiovascular exercise three times a week is sufficient to keep the heart healthy. Excessive cardiovascular exercise can also cause unnecessary stress to our joints, and this will eventually lead to chronic injury.

" ... take a look at the people working out with strength and resistance equipment. The people here are also training very hard. However, notice that the majority of them are in far better shape than the people in the cardiovascular section. So, in which section do you want to spend more time? "

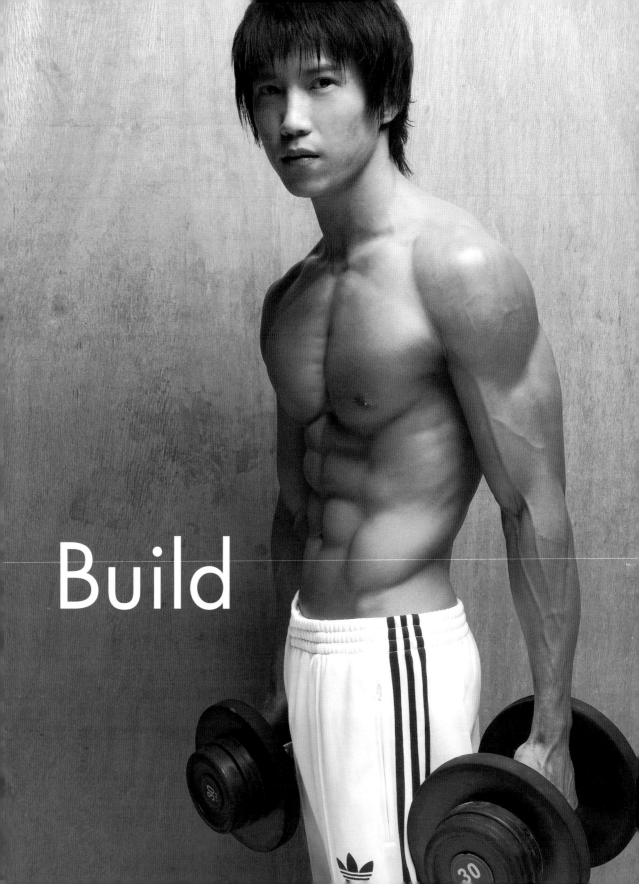

Build

Build

Besides helping us to lose body fat and gain muscle mass, strength and resistance training benefits our overall health in many ways.

Benefits of strength and resistance training

1. Higher calorie expenditure

As mentioned earlier, lean muscle tissue burns the most calories. When you weight-train, you build muscles. The end result is an increase in metabolism. This means that you will be enjoying the calorie-burning effect of cardiovascular exercise even when you are not working out. When you do cardiovascular exercise, you expend calories only during your exercise, but with weight training you burn additional calories 24 hours a day!

2. Greater physical strength

Weight training will increase your overall body strength. With this increased strength, many formerly physically stressful tasks will now seem much easier to overcome.

3. Lower likelihood of injury

As your muscles become stronger and more flexible, you will find that you are less prone to muscle sprains and muscle atrophy (muscle wasting).

4. Greater joint stability and flexibility

We will all experience some form of arthritis as we age. Strength and resistance training increases the strength in the tendons, ligaments and muscles surrounding our joints. This will put less stress on the joints, thus reducing the effects of arthritis.

5. Stronger lower back

When done correctly, strength and resistance training can strengthen your lower back, abdominals and muscles throughout your body. This will restore overall balance to your posture, and the end result is your lower back suffers less aches and pains.

6. Higher bone density and reduced risk of osteoporosis

Regular strength and resistance training is not just an exercise option; it is a necessity. Contrary to popular belief, repeated stress on the bones through strength and resistance training does not weaken them but actually strengthens them.

7. Decreased total serum cholesterol

Recent studies have shown that regular strength and resistance training reduces total cholesterol by 10 per cent and bad cholesterol, or low-density lipoprotein cholesterol (LDL), by as much as 14 per cent.

8. Reduced risk of Type II diabetes.

When muscle mass increases, the body is able to use insulin more efficiently. Insulin is a hormone that causes our bodies to transport sugar out of our blood, moving it to the tissues, where it is expended as energy.

9. Lower risk of colon cancer

Muscle building improves intestinal movement. The faster waste passes through the colon, the less likely carcinogens (cancer-causing substances) in faeces will attach to the intestinal wall, and this reduces our risk of developing colon cancer.

10. Lower risk of high blood pressure

A recent study cited by the American Heart Association's journal showed that in people who had gone through three months of strength and resistance training, systolic blood pressure (the force exerted against the artery walls during heart contraction) decreased by 2 per cent, and diastolic pressure (the force exerted on the artery walls during heart relaxation) fell by 4 per cent. This research indicates that the risk of getting heart disease and stroke may be reduced through resistance training.

11. Better posture and overall physical appearance

Properly executed strength and resistance training can significantly improve body posture. By developing certain muscles, we can all stand upright with our shoulders pulled back and abdomen tucked in. Our bodies will also appear more symmetrical.

12. Higher energy level

One study showed that participants who strength-trained for one year became 27 per cent more active, and their bodies became, on average, 15 to 20 years more youthful.

Repetitions, sets and your one repetition maximum (1RM)

There are three key terms that you will need to know before starting on a strength and resistance training programme:

Repetition: a repetition, or rep, refers to one complete exercise from start to finish.

Set: a set is a series of repetitions done without rest in between.

One repetition maximum (1RM): Your 1RM will differ from exercise to exercise. The 1RM is simply the maximum amount of weight you can carry for one repetition of an exercise. To determine your 1RM for an exercise, start with a weight you can comfortably carry to complete a repetition. Increase the weight by the smallest increment with each next repetition. Do this until you can no longer perform the exercise. The weight you carry on the last repetition is your 1RM.

For this programme, you will be doing sets of eight to ten repetitions at between 70 and 80 per cent of your 1RM. For beginners, I would recommend that they use lighter weights at the start of the programme. They should increase the weights progressively and only by the slightest increment. Do not rush to increase the weights as this may result in injury (this also applies to those who are more experienced).

When you do cardiovascular exercise, you expend calories only during your exercise, but with weight training you burn additional calories 24 hours a day!

Three essential components of a strength and resistance programme

1. Muscle isolation

There is an old weightlifter adage: "Link the mind to the muscle." Concentrate on the muscle you are working on. Studies have shown that the more you think about the muscle contracting and releasing while performing the exercise, the more you will stimulate and build the muscle fibre.

As you are performing a strength and resistance exercise, your muscle proceeds gradually to fatigue and then, ultimately, to failure. As you begin to tire the targeted muscle, other muscles will attempt to step in to assist the working muscle with the exercise. You do not want this to happen, as it will take the stress off the muscle you are trying to isolate and stimulate. In order to prevent this, concentrate on the muscle you are working and be conscious of keeping the correct form and posture.

2. Progressive overload

You must overload a muscle to force it to grow. Overloading means working your muscles to

their limits. A muscle is overloaded when it goes from fatigue to failure. If you can perform an exercise with ease, you are not overloading the muscle. The exercise has hit a plateau in terms of yielding results for your body, and you must apply new overload. Progressive overload is the gradual incorporation of other variables into your workout to ensure that your muscles do not get acclimatised to your exercises but have to continually work near their limits.

There are a number of variables you can adjust in your exercise regime to achieve progressive overload:

- Weight
  The simplest way to progress in your strength and resistance programme is to increase your training poundage or and tension (in simple terms, the weights you carry). Always add by the smallest weight increment.

  However, that does not mean that you must perform all repetitions with the heavier weights. Always start with the heavier weight, and as your muscle begins to go into fatigue and almost into failure, drop to a lower weight and perform the exercise to muscle failure.

- Repetitions
  With most of the exercises, I perform a maximum of 15 repetitions per set. After 15 repetitions, our joints may be at risk of injury. If you are not yet training at 15 repetitions, work till you get there. When

you reach 15, you will have to adjust one of the other variables.

- Sets

  As with repetitions, the number of sets you do at each gym session can also be increased. As the weeks go by, I progress from two sets per session to three and, finally, to four (see the programme plan on page 59). As long as you have not reached muscle failure, your muscle is not taxed fully and you can carry on.

- Speed

  Most people tend to neglect this aspect of progressive overload. You may start with a two-count positive motion (allowing yourself 2 seconds to lift the weight) followed by a two-count negative motion (taking 2 seconds to release the weight). To progressively overload, you could choose to go to a three-, four- or five-count speed. Many studies have shown that the safest and most effective way to stimulate a muscle is to do ten-count repetitions. But that is extremely difficult, and I cannot perform it on a regular basis.

- Angle

  Another way to advance your training is to change the angle at which you perform your exercises. Take the forward lunge as an example. Instead of lunging forwards and retracting backwards, which we will do initially, we could modify the movement by doing a 45-degree lunge. This means that, instead of stepping forwards directly, we step forwards at a 45-degree angle to the right or left. By doing this, other muscle groups, which ordinarily would not be worked when we perform the normal lunge, will be activated.

  Another example is the lat pulldown. We could change the angle in this exercise by changing the grip. Instead of having your palms facing down, why not have the palms facing up?

  However, I recommend that beginners do not change the angle of their exercises until they can successfully perform the exercises and isolate the muscle groups.

- Instability

  An exercise ball is a very good way to incorporate instability into an exercise. We stimulate more muscles by adding instability into our exercises. Let us take the dumbbell bench-press as an example. Normally, we lie down on a flat bench to perform this exercise. In doing so, we are stimulating the chest as the primary muscle, and the back of the arms as the secondary muscle. However, if we perform this exercise on an exercise ball, we also activate our abdominals and lower back muscles to maintain proper balance. In addition, our gluteus (rear end) muscles need to assist our body to stay up.

- Equipment

  If you have been using exercise machines to do your workout, you add progression by changing to free weights. Using free weights will activate more muscle groups for balance.

- Type of exercise
  Normally, a periodisation programme takes about eight weeks. In this period, I go on a programme where I push myself to the limit using a certain set of exercises. After this period, I will go off the programme and do other exercises, but not in a regimented way. After about eight weeks off the programme, I will start another programme using different exercises. In this way, my body will not get acclimatised to certain kinds of exercise, and routines for building muscle mass and reducing body fat will be more effective.

3. Breathing

Some people hold their breath when doing weight training. This is incorrect. Proper breathing techniques will allow us to lift heavier weights and work harder in the gym.

Keep these basic rules in mind:
- Exhale completely on exertion, or the difficult part of the exercise, and inhale completely as you release the weight. This will keep your body well oxygenated and enable you to perform more work during our exercise sessions.
- When lifting weights, remember to keep your mouth open to equalise the pressure in your chest.

Adapting the programme to your needs

I have to stress that this programme was designed specifically for me, and different people will respond differently to it. To make this programme work for you, modifications will have to be made to serve your specific needs.

> "You must overload a muscle to force it to grow.

Here are some pointers:

- Increase the intensity of the regime gradually, especially if you are a beginner. If you force yourself beyond your limits (such as carrying too heavy a weight), you will probably injure yourself and have to cease training.
- One size does not fit all. Understand your body and monitor the way it is responding to the programme. Fine-tune the programme to maximise your results and to minimise the risk of injury.
- Once you achieve your first target, adjust your routine to maintain your gains and start towards your next target.

The strength and resistance training programme

As you can see from the programme outline, on page 59, there are three weight training sessions scheduled each week. Remember to give yourself one or two days of rest after each session. Start by carrying 70 to 80 per cent of your 1RM for each exercise (see page 53). Beginners should start with lighter weights. Other important pointers:

- Perform the exercises in the order given in the programme.
- Perform a warm-up set, using slightly lighter weights, for all multi-joint exercises.
- Abdominal or core stability exercises should be performed in all your exercise sessions.
- For all exercises, exhale when you exert strength and inhale when releasing the weight.
- Rest 90 seconds in between sets.
- Do not sacrifice technique and form for a heavier weight.
- Stretch before and after each training session.

"Studies have shown that the more you think about the muscle contracting and releasing while performing the exercise, the more you will stimulate and build the muscle fibre.

Session 1	Week 1 Sets/repetitions	Week 2 Sets/repetitions	Week 3–10 Sets/repetitions
Dumbbell bench press	2 sets of 8	4 sets of 8	4 sets of 8
Squats	2 sets of 8	4 sets of 8	4 sets of 8
Chin ups	2 sets of 8	4 sets of 8	4 sets of 8
Dynamic dumbbell lunges	2 sets of 8	4 sets of 8	4 sets of 8
Standing dumbbell bicep curls	2 sets of 8	4 sets of 8	4 sets of 8
Reverse flyes	2 sets of 10	3 sets of 10	3 sets of 10
Standing woodchopper	2 sets of 10	3 sets of 10	3 sets of 10
Back extensions	2 sets of 10	3 sets of 10	3 sets of 10
Session 2	Week 1 Sets/repetitions	Week 2 Sets/repetitions	Week 3–10 Sets/repetitions
Incline bench press	2 sets of 8	4 sets of 8	4 sets of 8
Leg press	2 sets of 8	4 sets of 8	4 sets of 8
Seated dumbbell shoulder press	2 sets of 8	4 sets of 8	4 sets of 8
Seated row	2 sets of 8	4 sets of 8	4 sets of 8
Dumbbell flyes	2 sets of 8	4 sets of 8	4 sets of 8
Calf raises	2 sets of 15	3 sets of 15	3 sets of 15
Tricep pushdowns	2 sets of 8	4 sets of 8	4 sets of 8
Alternate arm and leg extensions	2 sets of 10	3 sets of 10	3 sets of 10
Session 3	Week 1 Sets/repetitions	Week 2 Sets/repetitions	Week 3–10 Sets/repetitions
Bench press	2 sets of 8	4 sets of 8	4 sets of 8
Squats	2 sets of 8	4 sets of 8	4 sets of 8
Lat pulldowns	2 sets of 8	4 sets of 8	4 sets of 8
45 degree dumbbell lunges	2 sets of 8	4 sets of 8	4 sets of 8
Barbell upright row	2 sets of 8	4 sets of 8	4 sets of 8
Standing reverse woodchopper	2 sets of 10	3 sets of 10	3 sets of 10
Back extensions	2 sets of 10	3 sets of 10	3 sets of 10
Exercises to be done at every session	Week 1 Sets/repetitions	Week 2 Sets/repetitions	Week 3–10 Sets/repetitions
Toe touches	3 sets of 20	3 sets of 20	3 sets of 20
Back extensions side bend	3 sets of 15	3 sets of 15	3 sets of 15
Lower abs	3 sets of 20	3 sets of 20	3 sets of 20
Gymnastic sit-ups	3 sets of 25	3 sets of 25	3 sets of 25
Static hold (front and side)	Hold for 30 secs	Hold for 30 secs	Hold for 30 secs

Session 1

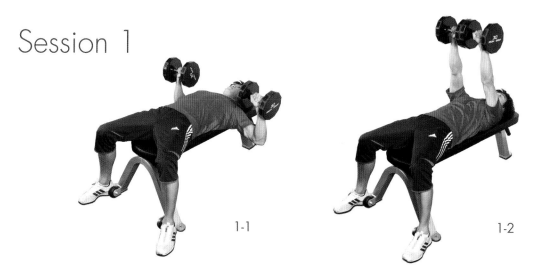

1-1

1-2

1. Dumbbell Bench Press

a.   Lie on the bench with a dumbbell in each hand (picture 1-1).

b.   Exhaling, slowly lift the dumbbells over your chest (picture 1-2). Concentrate on pushing your chest muscles as you perform the exercise.

c.   Inhaling, slowly lower the dumbbells back to the starting position.

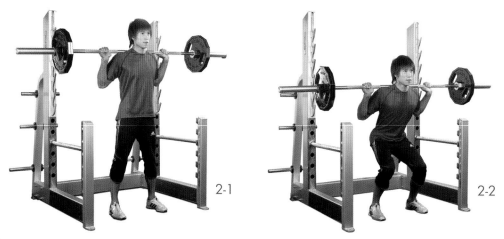

2-1

2-2

2. Squats

a.   Stand upright with your feet about shoulder-width apart. Rest the barbell on your upper back (picture 2-1).

b.   Slowly bend your legs and lower your buttocks until your thighs are parallel to the floor (picture 2-2). To help keep your back straight, try tilting your head up and looking straight at the ceiling.

c.   Return to the starting position.

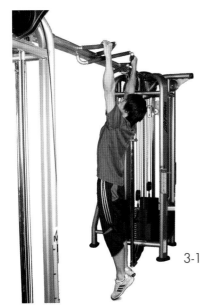

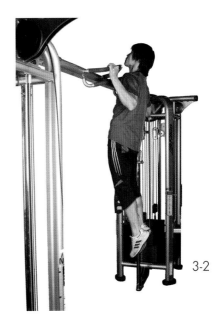

3-1

3-2

3. Chin Ups

a. Get into position as shown in picture 3-1. Hold the bar with an overhand grip (your palms facing outwards).

b. Exhaling, pull yourself up until your chin is above the bar. Concentrate on squeezing the back muscles as you lift yourself up (picture 3-2).

c. Lower yourself to the starting position.

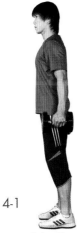

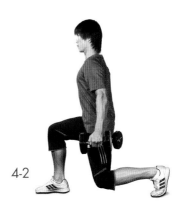

4-1

4-2

4. Dynamic Dumbbell Lunges

a. Stand up straight, holding a dumbbell in each hand (picture 4-1).

b. Step your right foot forwards, bending both knees until your right thigh is parallel to the floor (picture 4-2). Keep your back straight at all times.

c. Return to the starting position.

d. Repeat the exercise with the left leg.

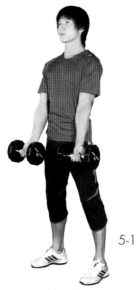

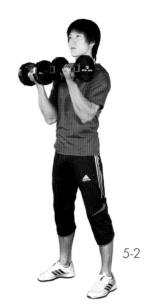

5-1

5-2

5. Standing Dumbbell Bicep Curls

a. Stand upright with a dumbbell in each hand (picture 5-1).

b. Exhaling, slowly raise the dumbbells to your chest (picture 5-2). Keep your elbows tucked to your side.

c. Inhale, as you lower the dumbbells to the starting position.

d. You can choose to lift both dumbbells at the same time or alternate between each hand.

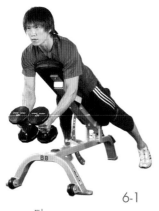

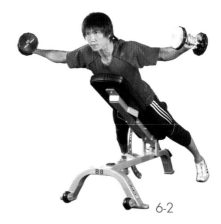

6-1

6-2

6. Reverse Flyes

a. With a dumbbell in each hand, rest on an inclined bench (picture 6-1).

b. Slowly raise the dumbbells out to the sides (picture 6-2), exhaling at the same time. Bend your elbows and wrists slightly. Concentrate on squeezing the back of your shoulders.

c. When you have lifted the dumbbells to shoulder height, slowly lower the dumbbells to the starting position.

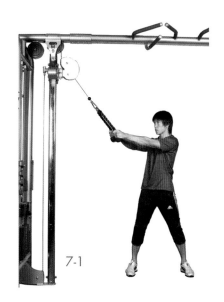

7-1

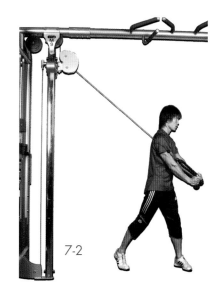

7-2

7. Standing Woodchopper

a. Stand at the machine with feet shoulder-width apart (picture 7-1).

b. Pull the handle diagonally across your chest and down to waist level (picture 7-2). While performing this step, rotate your torso using strength from your stomach as well. Keep your elbows slightly bent.

c. Return to the starting position slowly.

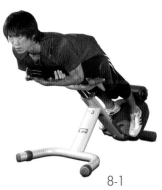

8-1

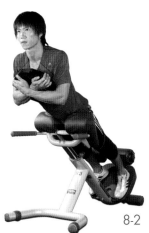

8-2

8. Back Extensions

a. Position yourself on the back extension machine as shown in picture 8-1. Do not extend your hip joint above the pad as this will take the focus off your lower back. Relax your back and keep your legs straight.

b. Exhale as you straighten your spine slowly, raising your head, your upper torso and then your back, as shown in picture 8-2.

c. Hold this position for one second and then slowly return to the starting position. Inhale as you lower your body.

d. At a more advanced level, try holding a weight while performing this exercise.

Session 2

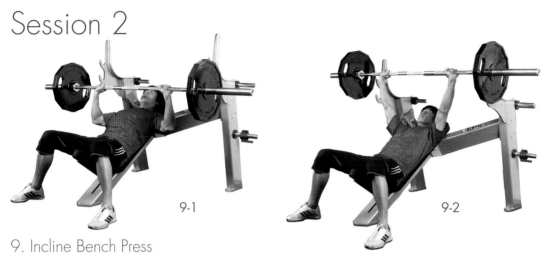

9-1

9-2

9. Incline Bench Press

a. Lie on the incline bench and grip the bar; your hands should be slightly more than shoulder-width apart.
b. Lift the barbell slowly and extend your arms fully.
c. Lower the barbell just over the lower part of your chest (picture 9-1).
d. Exhaling, begin pushing the barbell up until your arms are fully extended again (picture 9-2).
e. Inhaling, lower the barbell to starting position.

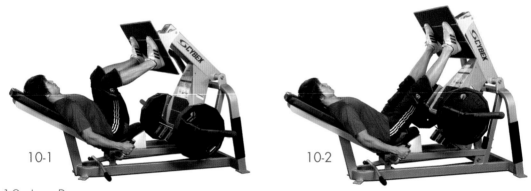

10-1

10-2

10. Leg Press

a. Position yourself on the leg press machine as shown in picture 10-1 and place your feet about 15 to 30 centimetres apart on the platform.
b. Release the safety catch on the machine and let your legs bear the weight. Lower the platform to the starting position as shown in picture 10-1.
c. Slowly lift the weights by straightening your legs. Exhale as you do so (picture 10-2).
d. Just before your legs are fully extended, bend your legs back to the starting position. Inhale as you do so.

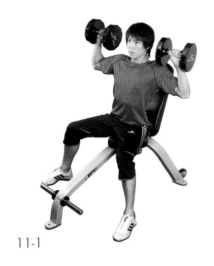

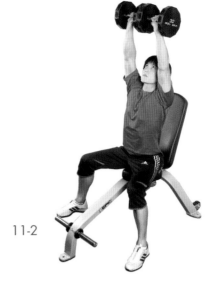

11-1

11-2

11. Seated Dumbbell Shoulder Press

a. Sitting with your back straight, hold a pair of dumbbells over your shoulders as shown in picture 11-1.
b. Exhaling slowly, extend your arms until the dumbbells are above your head as shown in picture 11-2. Concentrate on squeezing your shoulders as you perform the exercise.
c. Return the dumbbell to the starting position, inhaling at the same time.

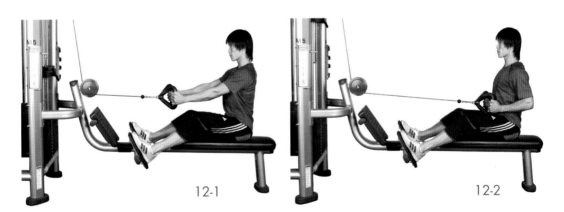

12-1

12-2

12. Seated Row

a. Sit upright on the bench of the seated row machine, grasping hold of the cable handle (picture 12-1).
b. Remember to keep your knees bent and your back straight and perpendicular to the bench. Exhaling, pull the cable handle to your upper abdominal area (picture 12-2). Do not move your torso, only your arms should move.
c. Hold the contraction for a second before slowly returning to the starting position. Inhale as you straighten your arms.

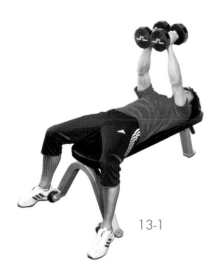

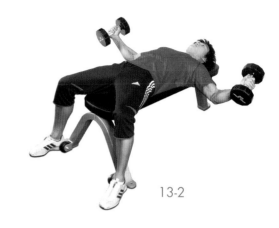

13-1

13-2

13. Dumbbell Flyes

a. Lie back on a bench with a dumbbell in each hand. Extend your arms fully above your chest (picture 13-1).
b. Lower the dumbbells down to the sides (picture 13-2). You should be able to feel the stretch on your chest as you lower the weights. Keep your elbows slightly bent as your perform this exercise.
c. When the dumbbells are level with your body, slowly lift the weights back to the starting position, squeezing your chest as you do so.

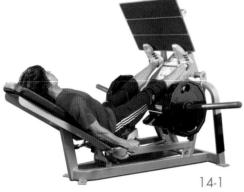

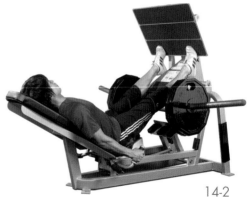

14-1

14-2

14. Calf Raises

a. On the leg press machine, fully extend your legs with only your toes and the balls of your feet in contact with the edge of the platform.
b. Release the catch on the machine and let your legs bear the weight (picture 14-1).
c. Locking your knees and using only your ankles, lift the platform by pushing your toes forwards (picture 14-2).
d. Return the platform to the starting position.

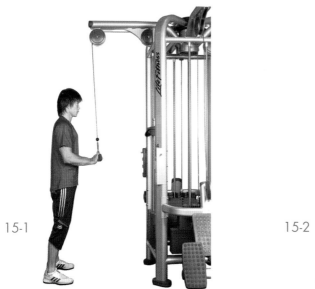
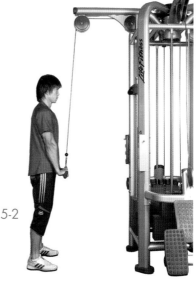

15-1 15-2

15. Triceps Pushdowns

a. Stand in front of a triceps pushdown bar with your feet shoulder-width apart. Grasp the bar with palms facing down (picture 15-1).

b. Lean slightly forwards and push the bar down while keeping the upper arms stationary (picture 15-2).

c. Remember to use only your forearms to push the bar down.

d. When your forearms are straightened, return the bar to the starting position.

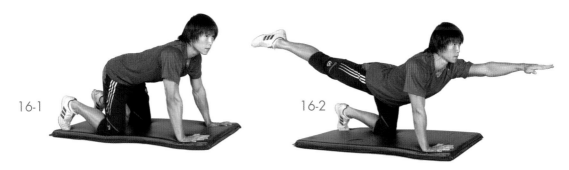

16-1 16-2

16. Alternate Arm and Leg Extensions

a. Position your hands and knees shoulder-width apart on the floor (picture 16-1).

b. Slowly exhale as you lift your left arm and right leg up (picture 16-2). Hold, keeping your chin down and your stomach tucked in. Concentrate on your back muscles as you lift and squeeze them.

c. Inhale as you return to the starting position.

d. Repeat with your right arm and left leg.

Session 3

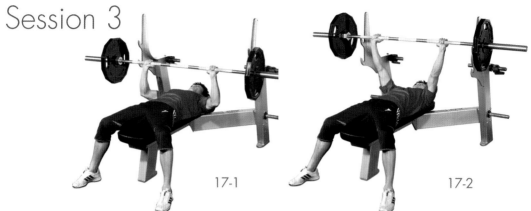

17-1   17-2

17. Bench Press

a. Lie on the bench and grip the bar; your arms should be slightly more than shoulder-width apart.

b. Lift the barbell slowly and extend your arms fully.

c. Lower the barbell slowly to your chest, keeping it just over the lower part of your chest (picture 17-1). This is the starting position.

d. Exhaling, begin pushing the barbell up until your arms are fully extended again (picture 17-2).

e. Inhale as you lower the barbell to the starting position.

18. Squats (see exercise 2.)

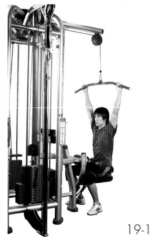

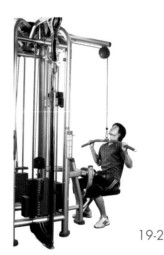

19-1   19-2

19. Lat Pulldowns

a. Hold on to the bar with a wide pronated grip (palms facing away from your body) as shown in picture 19-1.

b. Exhale as you pull down the bar to your upper chest (picture 19-2).

c. Inhale as you return the bar to the overhead position.

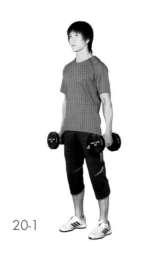

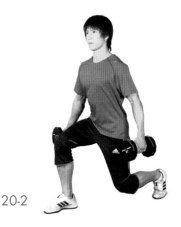

20-1

20-2

20. 45-degree Dumbbell Lunges

This exercise is similar to the Dynamic Dumbbell Lunges except that, instead of stepping straight ahead, you step 45 degrees to your side.

a.   Stand upright and hold the dumbbells by your side (picture 20-1).

b.   Step forwards 45 degrees to your side with one leg, bending your knees, as shown in picture 20-2, until both thighs are parallel to the floor. Keep your back straight.

c.   Return to the starting position and repeat with the other leg.

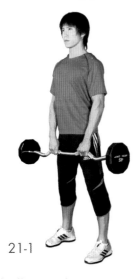

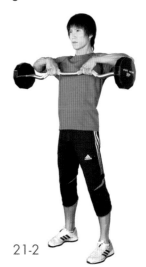

21-1

21-2

21. Barbell Upright Row

a.   Hold on to the barbell with your arms fully extended downwards (picture 21-1).

b.   Exhaling slowly, lift the barbell upwards (in line with your body) until it reaches above your upper chest (picture 21-2). Keep your elbows above the level of your palms throughout this exercise.

c.   Slowly lower the bar to the starting position, inhaling at the same time.

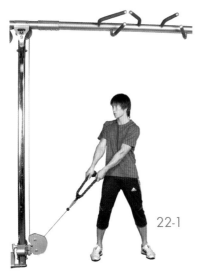

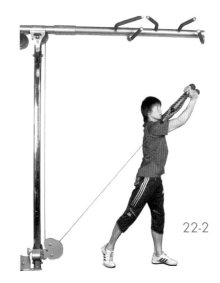

22-1

22-2

22. Standing Reverse Woodchopper

a. Stand at the woodchopper machine with your legs shoulder width-apart (picture 22-1).

b. Pull the handle up from the right across your chest until it is above your head on the left (picture 22-2). As you pull, rotate your torso using your stomach muscles. Keep your elbows slightly bent as you perform the exercise.

c. Slowly return to the starting position.

23. Back Extensions (see exercise 8.)

Exercises to be performed at every session

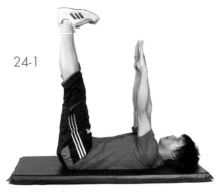

24-1

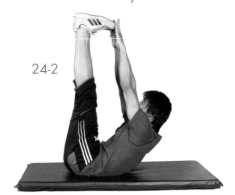

24-2

24. Toe Touches

a. Lie on your back. Raise your legs until they are perpendicular to the floor (picture 24-1).

b. Extend your arms and reach for your toes (picture 24-2), contracting your stomach muscles as you do so.

c. Return to the starting position.

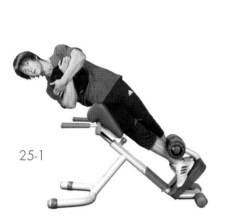 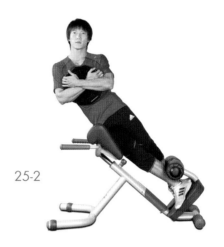

25-1   25-2

25. Back Extensions Side Bend

a. Get into position at the machine as shown in picture 25-1.

b. Do not extend your hip joint over the pad as this will take the focus away from your lower back and obliques (the sides of your stomach). Concentrate on using your obliques as you perform the exercise. Relax your back and keep your legs straight.

c. Straighten your spine slowly, raising your head, then your upper torso and then your back (picture 25-2). Exhale as you perform this step.

d. Hold this position for a second and then slowly return to the starting position. Inhale as you lower your body. When you have mastered the basic movements of this exercise, you may wish to carry a weight performing it.

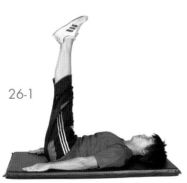 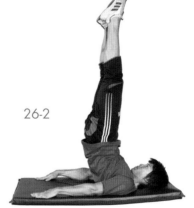

26-1   26-2

26. Lower Abs

a. Lie down on your back with your legs raised as shown in picture 26-1.

b. Flex your stomach muscles to lift your back off the floor until you get into the position shown in picture 26-2.

c. Return your legs to the starting position.

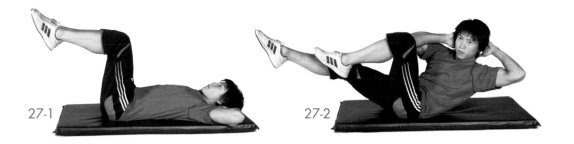

27-1   27-2

27. Gymnastic Sit-ups

a. Assume the position shown in picture 27-1.
b. Bring your right elbow and your left knee together, as shown in picture 27-2, focusing your effort on contracting your abdominal muscles.
c. Return to the starting position and repeat with your left elbow and your right knee.

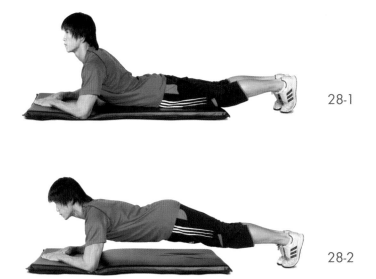

28-1

28-2

28. Static Hold: Front

a. Assume the position shown in picture 28-1.
b. Squeeze your stomach muscles as you slowly lift your body off the floor (picture 28-2). Hold this position for 30 seconds, keeping your stomach muscles contracted. While in this position, breathe using your chest muscles instead of your diaphragm.
c. Return to the starting position.

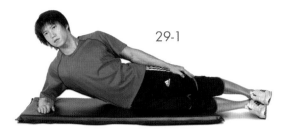 29-1

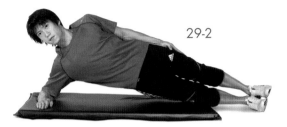 29-2

29. Static Hold: Side

a. Assume the position shown in picture 29-1.

b. Contract your oblique muscles as you lift your body off the floor (picture 29-2). Hold this position for 30 seconds, keeping your obliques contracted. Breathe using your chest muscles instead of your diaphragm.

c. Repeat the exercise.

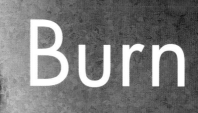

Burn

Burn

Our heart is the single most important muscle in our body, and performing cardiovascular exercises will help preserve it. By strengthening our heart, we can prevent many heart-related problems, like high-blood pressure, stroke and heart attack.

When we train aerobically, by swimming, jogging, walking or cycling, for example, we raise our heart rates and so increase our bodies' consumption of oxygen. This not only benefits the heart and lungs and improves circulation, but also increases the rate at which we burn calories for the duration of the exercise. The table below lists the approximate number of calories burned during 30 minutes of different physical activities.

Type of activity	60-kg adult	80-kg adult
Walking	130	180
Cycling	180	240
Swimming	210	300
Jogging	300	400
In-line skating	210	280
Aerobic dance	180	240
Singles tennis	180	270
Frisbee	180	240
Skiing	240	330
Weightlifting	210	240

When we are active, our bodies burn fat and sugar. However, when we are less fit our bodies burn more sugar than fat. This means that as we become fitter, the ability of our bodies to burn fat will increase as well.

For our bodies to burn fat most efficiently, we need to train within our optimum training zone. What this means is that we have to do exercises that will cause our hearts to beat at the rate specified in the optimum training zone. This zone is generally between 75 and 90 per cent of the individual's maximum heart rate. Beginners should target a heart rate of between 60 and 75 per cent of their maximum heart rate; intermediate exercisers should target 75 to 80 per cent; and advanced exercisers should aim for 85 to 90 per cent.

Maximum Heart Rate

An individual's maximum heart rate is calculated as follows:

220 – individual's age = maximum heart rate

My maximum heart rate:
220 – 31 = 189 beats per minute

The easiest way to monitor our heart rate during exercise is to wear a heart rate monitor. Alternatively, we could take our pulse for 15 seconds and multiply it by four.

The higher the intensity of the workout, the higher your heart rate, and this means that more fat will be burned. To enhance the fat-burning effects of your workouts, do them in the morning while your body is in a fasted state.

Progression

The same concept of progression that we use in strength and resistance training applies to cardiovascular exercise. We can vary our workouts by speed, frequency and intensity.

Even in a single session, incorporating progression can greatly enhance its fat burning effect. When running, for example, I begin by warming up for 2 minutes, performing at 50 per cent of my maximum speed. Then I take it up a notch to 60 per cent for a minute. I increase my speed by 10 per cent after every minute until I reach 90 per cent of my maximum speed. After doing 90 per cent for a minute, I will bring it down to 60 per cent again. Excluding the warm-up phase, the whole cycle (from 60 to 90 per cent) takes 4 minutes.

I repeat this cycle three more times. However, in the last cycle, I do not stop at 90 per cent. Instead, I try to aim for 100 per cent for a minute, before bringing it all the way back to 50 per cent for 2 minutes (cooling down). By doing this, I confuse my body and this ensures that it will not get used to the activity level.

In this way, my body is constantly working hard to burn fat.

The cardiovascular exercise plan

I devote 25 per cent of my workout time on cardiovascular exercise. You might like to incorporate this into your weight training sessions or perform it on the days you are away from the gym.

The type of cardiovascular exercise that you choose to do is up to you, but it will be more effective if you were to incorporate the element of progression I outlined above. Personally, I prefer wushu, rollerblading and wakeboarding.

"The higher the intensity of the workout, the higher your heart rate, and this means that more fat will be burned. To enhance the fat-burning effects of your workouts, do your workouts in the morning while your body is in a fasted state.

Flexibility is an often neglected but important component of fitness. By stretching before and after training, we ensure that our muscles are elastic. Muscles that are more pliant pack more power, as they are able to contract and extend to a greater degree. If our muscles become tight and inflexible, blood flow becomes impaired, which in turn disrupts muscle contraction and function. If a chronically tense muscle is left untreated, it will eventually cause problems in our spine and joints. Therefore, stretching a muscle to improve flexibility is essential. Stretching in between routines also gives us greater stamina in our workouts as it decreases muscle fatigue. It can also help prevent injuries.

The main aims of warming up are to raise the body temperature, to limber up the muscles and connective tissues, and to increase blood circulation. I like to spend about half an hour to an hour warming up. I begin with about 10 minutes of light jogging followed by stretching exercises. After the workout, I spend another half an hour to cool down. Doing stretching exercises after the workout will aid in the recovery process; the muscles will not feel so sore the next day. It will also ensure that muscles remain elastic and can generate more power. This is very essential in wushu, where flexibility and muscle power are crucial to peak performance.

Another way of cooling down is to go for a massage. A good massage therapist will work the muscles to relieve the tension, releasing muscle adhesions (scar tissue) that are locking the muscle fibres together.

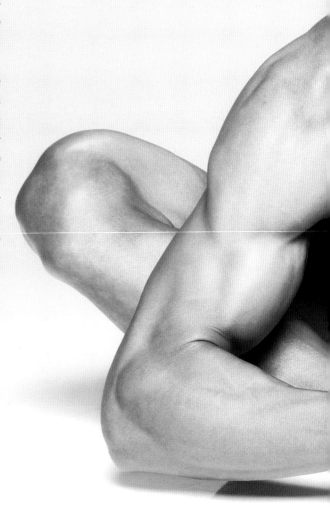

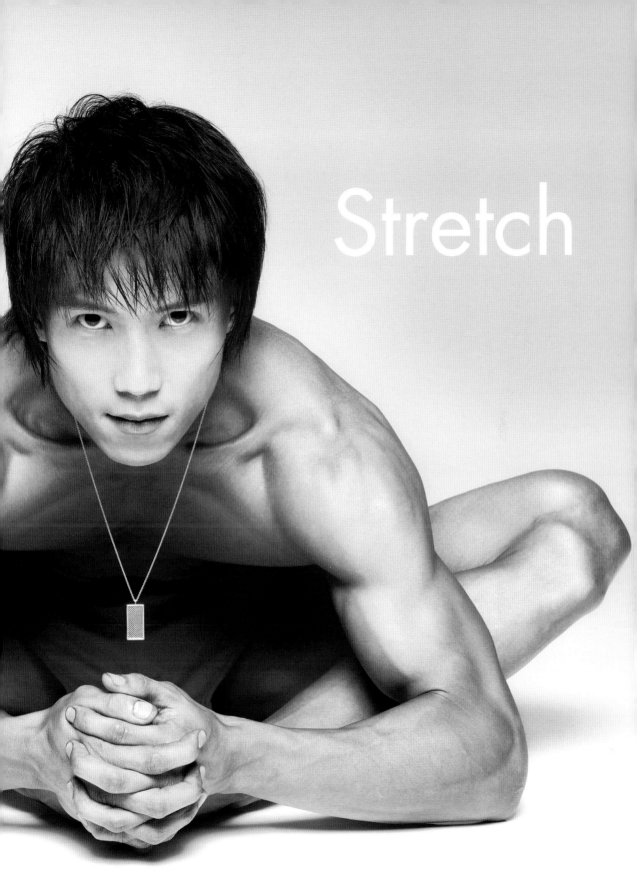

Stretch

"Muscles that are more pliant pack more power, as they are able to contract and extend to a greater degree.„

Stretching exercises

The following are some stretching exercises that I regularly perform. Do incorporate them before and after each weight training or cardiovascular exercise sessions.

Upper body stretches

Front of shoulder

- Stand upright with your right side near the wall and place your right hand against the wall at shoulder level, such that your arm is perpendicular to the wall. Straighten your arm. Slowly turn your body away from the wall, feeling the stretch in your forearms, biceps, front shoulder and chest. Repeat with your other arm.

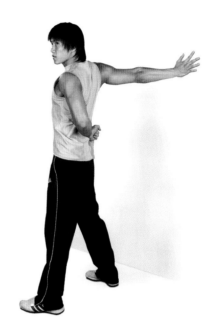

Back of shoulder

- Standing upright, position your arms behind your back with both hands locked together. Start with your elbows fully extended and your hands resting on your buttocks. From this position, slowly raise both arms as high as possible while maintaining your upright posture. If you cannot get your hands to meet at your back, try grasping a rolled-up towel.

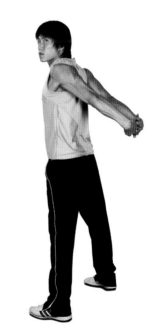

Back of shoulder (single arm)

- Bring one arm over your chest, parallel with the floor, until you feel a stretch in the rear shoulder area. Repeat with the other arm.

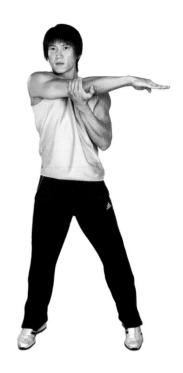

Triceps

- Start by raising both arms above your head. Then bend your right elbow and hold it with your left hand. Slowly try to reach farther down your back with your right hand. Repeat with your left elbow.

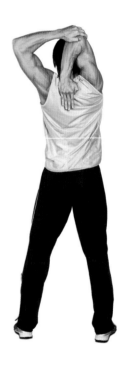

Spine

- Stand upright with your knees slightly bent and feet hip-width apart. Cross your arms in front of you and raise them to shoulder level. Without moving your hips, rotate your upper body to one side. Hold for 6 to 8 seconds and then rotate to the other side.

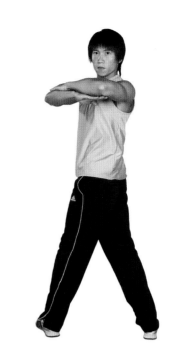

Upper back

- Stand with your feet hip-width apart, knees slightly bent. Interlock your fingers and position your hands in front of you. Your arms should be raised to shoulder level. Keeping your elbows slightly bent, stretch your arms, pushing your hands out in front of you. Hold the position for 8 to 10 seconds.

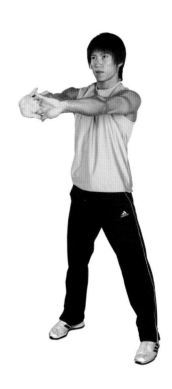

Lower body stretches

Calf

- Stand facing a wall. Lean your upper body forwards, placing your palms on the wall for support. Your arms, back and legs should be kept straight as shown in the picture. You should feel a stretch in your calves. Step your right leg forwards to increase the stretch in your left calf; your heel should be on the ground when you do this. Hold for 10 seconds. Repeat with the left leg.

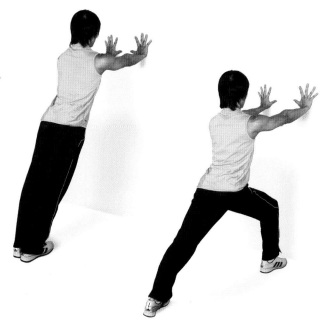

Quadriceps

- Using a wall for support, lift your left foot up behind you and hold it with your left hand. Slowly pull your left foot back against your buttocks to stretch the left quadriceps. Repeat with the right leg.

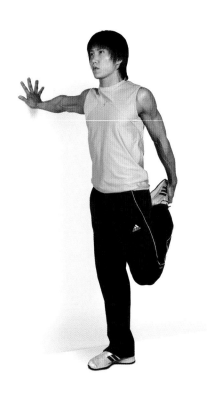

Hip flexor lunge

- Starting in a standing position, lunge forwards with your left leg, keeping the right leg back with the knee bent. Resting your hands on the ground, your left leg should be kept perpendicular to the floor as you lower the trunk of your body and position it as far forwards as possible. You should feel the stretch in the groin area. Repeat with the other leg.

Hamstring (single leg)

- Start in a sitting position with your right leg extended forwards and your left leg bent. Rest the sole of your left foot on your inner right thigh. Keep your right leg straight as you lean forwards as far as you can, reaching for your right ankle, heel or toes. Repeat with the other leg.

Hamstring (double leg) and inner groin

- In a sitting position, straighten your legs and spread them apart. Keep your arms shoulder-width apart and rest them in a U-shape as shown in the picture. Next, bring your arms together, lower your upper body and reach forwards till your face is almost to the floor.

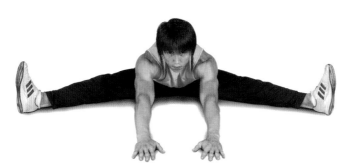

Groin

- Bring the soles of your feet together and lean your body forwards. Rest your elbows on your lower legs and grasp your feet with both hands. Continue to lean forwards until you feel the stretch in your groin area.

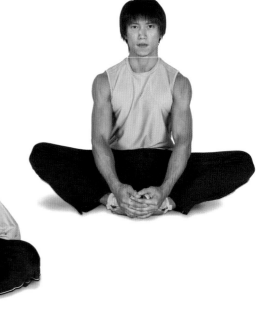

Spinal twist

- Sit with your legs fully extended. Place your right leg over your left leg, keeping your left leg straight and your right knee bent. Rest your left elbow on your right knee and twist your upper body to the right, using your left arm to assist in the twisting motion. Repeat on the other side.

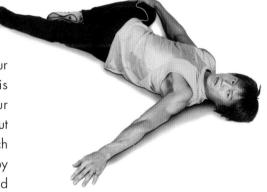

Lower back

- Start by lying on your back. Position your left leg over your right leg so that it is perpendicular to your body. Keep your shoulders flat on the floor and your arms out to the sides. You should feel a gentle stretch in your lower back. Increase the stretch by grasping your left leg with your right hand and pulling your left knee towards the floor. Repeat with the other leg.

Home Workouts

There may be times when you are unable to get to the gym for your workouts. Although it may be difficult to use the exercises featured here to yield significant progress as most of us do not have the heavier weights available at a well-equipped gym, these exercises can help maintain your form until your next gym workout.

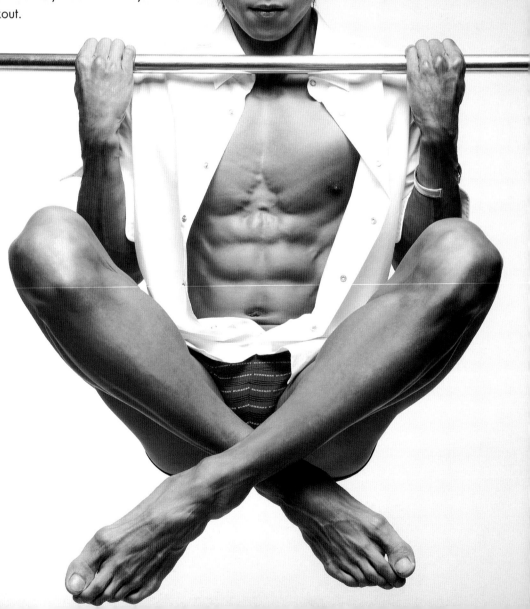

"Although it may be difficult to use the (home) exercises featured here to yield significant progress ... these exercises can help maintain your form until your next gym workout.

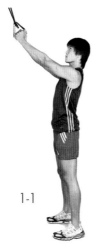

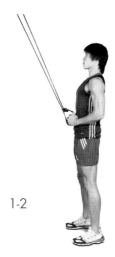

1-1

1-2

1. Lat pulldowns (works the back)

a. Attach the elastic tube to a high railing.

b. Adopt the position shown in picture 1-1.

c. Slowly exhale as you pull the handles down (picture 1-2). Concentrate on your back muscles, squeezing them at the end of this movement. Keep your shoulder and neck muscles relaxed throughout the exercise.

d. Inhale as you release the handles back to the starting position.

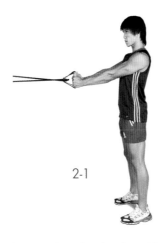

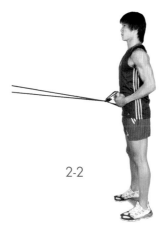

2-1

2-2

2. Back row (works the back)

a. Attach the elastic tube to a firm railing that is at waist level.

b. Adopt the standing position as shown in picture 2-1

c. Slowly exhale as you pull your elbows in as shown in picture 2-2. Inhale as you release the tubes back to the starting position.

d. Concentrate on your back muscles, squeezing them at the end of the exertion.

e. Keep your shoulder and neck muscles relaxed at all times.

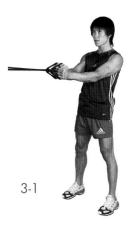

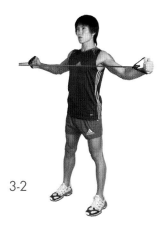

3-1

3-2

3. Rear deltoid flyes (works the back of the shoulders)

a. Attach the elastic tube to a firm railing at chest level.

b. Adopt the position shown in picture 3-1.

c. Exhale slowly as you pull your arms back and away from each other (picture 3-2). Keep your elbows slightly bent and your shoulder and neck relaxed throughout the exercise. Concentrate on the back of your shoulders as you pull on the handles.

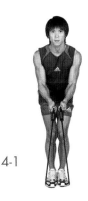

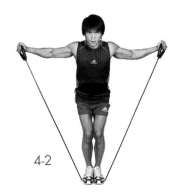

4-1

4-2

4. Standing lateral raise (works the middle deltoid or mid-shoulders)

a. Secure the elastic tube under your feet and adopt the position shown in picture 4-1.

b. Lean forwards slightly to isolate the middle part of your shoulders.

c. Exhale slowly as you pull the handles up to the sides until they reach shoulder level (picture 4-2). Keep your elbows slightly bent and your shoulder and neck relaxed throughout the exercise. Concentrate on the middle deltoid as you pull on the tube.

d. Release and lower your arms to the starting position.

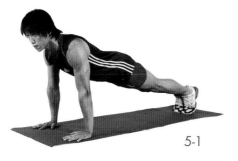 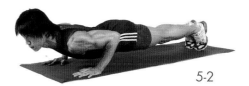

5-1 5-2

5. Push-ups (works the chest and triceps)

a. Adopt the position shown in picture 5-1. Your hands should be shoulder-width apart and your fingers spread out.

b. If you are a beginner, support your legs with your knees. If you are stronger, use your toes or you could even elevate your legs.

c. Inhale slowly as you lower yourself down as shown in picture 5-2. Exhale as you bring yourself up.

d. Concentrate on your chest at all times, especially when you lift yourself up. Keep your abdomen tucked in at all times to support your lower back.

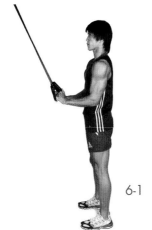 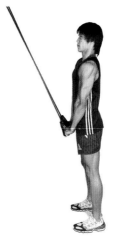

6-1 6-2

6. Triceps push-downs (works the back of the arms)

a. Attach the elastic tube to a firm high railing.

b. Adopt the standing position shown in picture 6-1, tucking your elbows to your sides.

c. Exhale slowly as you bring the handles down (picture 6-2).

d. Inhale when you release the tube to the starting position. When executing this exercise, concentrate your effort on the back of your arms, squeezing them at the end of the exertion. Keep your shoulder and neck muscles relaxed at all times.

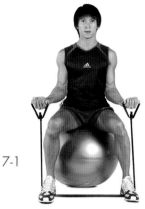

7-1

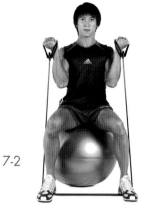

7-2

7. Bicep curls sitting on the ball (works the front of the arms)

a. Sit on an exercise ball with the elastic tube under your feet (picture 7-1).

b. Exhale slowly as you pull the tube handles up to chest level, (picture 7-2). Concentrate on your biceps, the front part of the arm, as you lift the handles. Keep your elbows to your sides throughout the exercise.

c. When the handles reach shoulder-level, release the elastic tube to the starting position. Inhale as you release.

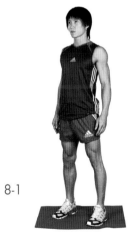

8-1

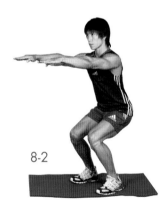

8-2

8. Squats (works the lower body)

a. Adopt the position shown in picture 8-1. Your toes should be pointing forwards, your abdomen tucked in and your back straightened.

b. Slowly inhale as you squat down until your thighs are parallel to the floor (picture 8-2).

c. Exhale as you lift yourself up, concentrating on squeezing your rear end.

d. Do not move your knees beyond your toes. Try to sit yourself farther back to prevent this from happening.

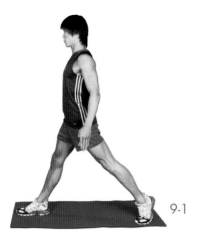
9-1

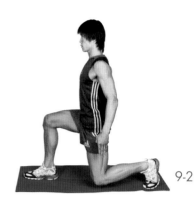
9-2

9. Stationary lunges (works the lower body)

a. Put your right foot forwards and your left foot back as shown in picture 9-1.

b. Inhale slowly as you lower your body, bending both knees (picture 9-2). Concentrate on squeezing your rear end as you perform the exercise. Keep your stomach tucked in and do not lean forwards. Your right knee should not move beyond your right foot.

c. Exhale as you slowly lift yourself back to the starting position.

d. Repeat the exercise with the other leg.

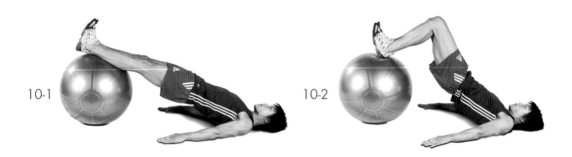
10-1   10-2

10. Hamstring curls on an exercise ball (works the back of the thighs)

a. Lie on your back with your legs propped up on the exercise ball (picture 10-1).

b. Make sure your stomach is tucked in and your neck is relaxed.

c. Slowly exhale as you pull your heels towards you (picture 10-2). Hold this position at the end of this movement and squeeze the muscles at the back of your thighs. Keep your legs aligned at all times.

d. As you return to the starting position, inhale.

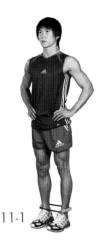

11-1

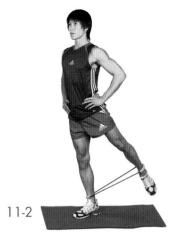

11-2

11. Hip extensions (works the hip and back the thighs)

a. Place the elastic loop around your ankles (picture 11-1).
b. Exhale slowly as you move your left leg behind you until the elastic loop is at its maximum tension (picture 11-2). Concentrate on your rear as you squeeze the leg back during the exertion phase.
c. Inhale as you return to the starting position.
d. Repeat the exercise with the other leg.

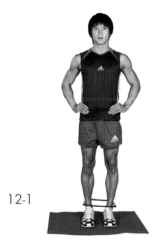

12-1

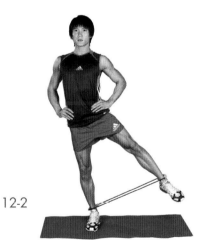

12-2

12. Hip abductions (works the outer thighs, abductor muscle and hips)

a. Place the elastic loop around your ankles (picture 12-1).
b. Exhale slowly as you move your left leg out to your side. Stop only when the loop is at its maximum tension (picture 12-2). Concentrate on your outer thigh.
c. Inhale as you return to the starting position.
d. Repeat the exercise with the other leg.

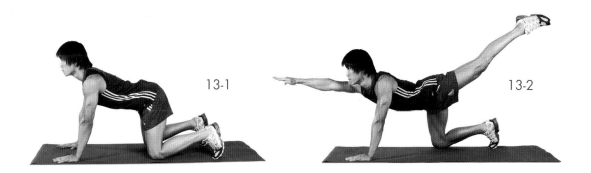

13. Back extensions (works the lower back)

a. Position yourself on your hands and knees as shown in picture 13-1. Your back should be straight and your arms and legs should be shoulder-width apart.

b. Simultaneously lift your right arm and your left leg up in the air as shown in picture 13-2. Hold this position for as long as you can, keeping your chin down and your stomach tucked in. Concentrate on your back.

c. Pause for a moment and inhale as you return to the starting position.

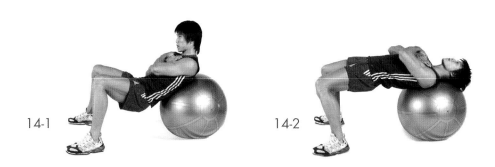

14. Bridging the ball (works the lower back)

a. Rest your shoulders on the ball as shown in picture 14-1. Start with your rear end relaxed and positioned lower than your chest.

b. Exhale slowly as you lift your rear end and lower back until you assume the position shown in picture 14-2. Concentrate on squeezing your rear end and lower back. At the end of the movement, your upper body and thighs should be parallel with the floor.

c. Pause for a moment and inhale as you return to the starting position.

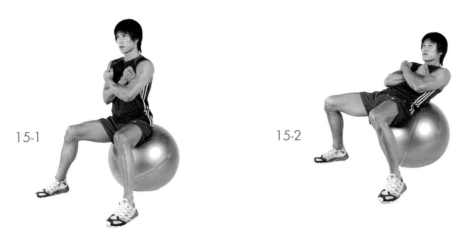

15-1

15-2

15. Abdominals (works the stomach)

a. Sit on an exercise ball. Your feet should be shoulder-width apart and your toes pointing forwards (picture 15-1).

b. Lean back and concentrate on focusing the tension on your abdominal muscles (picture 15-2).

c. Exhale slowly as you lift your body about 7 cm above the ball. If you feel pain in your back, stop the exercise immediately.

d. Inhale as you lower your body to starting position.

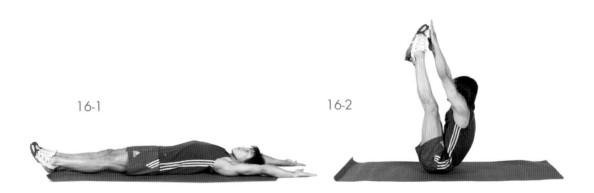

16-1

16-2

16. Abdominals 2 (works the upper and lower stomach)

a. Lie flat on the floor with your hands fully extended above your head (picture 16-1).

b. Exhale slowly as you bring your arms and legs together in mid-air (picture 16-2).

c. Concentrate on squeezing your stomach muscles.

d. Return to the starting position.

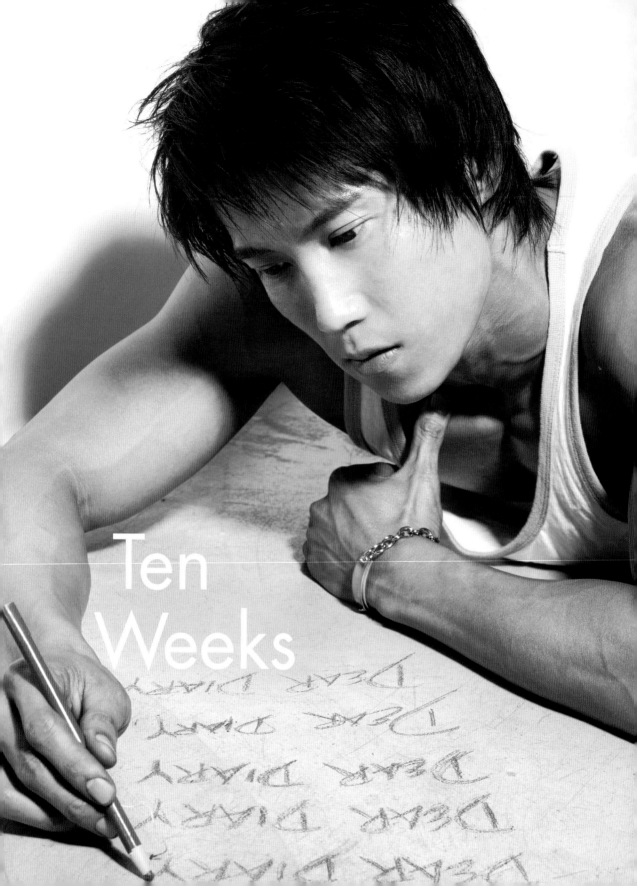

Ten
Weeks

DEAR DIARY
DEAR DIARY
DEAR DIARY
DEAR DIARY
DEAR DIARY

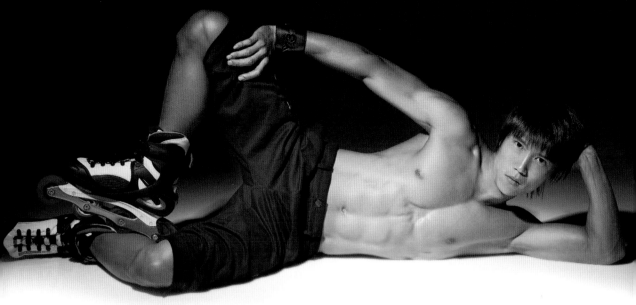

Vincent's Ten Weeks
WEEK 1

This week was the warm-up phase of the programme. I was motivated and excited. As I had not many work commitments this week, all my workouts were duly completed (I trained on Monday, Wednesday and Friday; each session lasted 2 hours). In fact, I even had enough time to rollerblade and have coffee with my friends.

With the help of the Singapore Sports Council, I was given permission to do my workouts at the Kallang Athlete Training Centre. This was my first time in this gym since I left the national wushu team, and I had to get used to the machines and weights again. I had to determine the maximum weight I could carry on each machine. Perhaps it is just my poor memory but I distinctly remember being able to lift heavier weights when I last trained at the sports centre.

The Kallang Athlete Training Centre is for exclusive use by national athletes and, naturally, it is the best equipped of the Sports Council gyms. The national wushu team used to train here once a week, as it did not have a fully equipped gym of its own back then. Coming here again reminded me of the time I spent training here with my teammates, a time when I was still representing Singapore. I remember how I would be working on a machine, totally drenched with sweat, while my coach stood by my side, encouraging me to work even harder. I really do have many fond memories of this place.

The training programme designed by James Wong, the head of strength and conditioning at the Singapore Sports Council, is very comprehensive. It ensures that I get an almost full body workout every week and it is very enjoyable. When I trained on my own, I only worked the parts of the body that were of benefit to my wushu routines. Although I trained myself to the limit this week, I felt that this was still far below what I used to be able to do. I am really looking forward to doing better soon.

I found the nutrition plan to be quite easy to follow. The diet is quite varied and I did not get sick of my meals. I have to admit that I eat almost anything and have a voracious appetite. Yet I was in control this week. Maybe it was the 'eating spree' I went on before I started on the programme.

My mother cooks for the family very often. However, I could not have my meals at home this week. I felt really bad, as she had spent a lot of time and effort cooking. This was partly my fault, as I did not give her the specifics of my diet. I did mention to her that I was following a nutrition plan and that I wanted her to cook healthy food for me. But my mother has a different idea of what is healthy. To her,

porridge with deep-fried chicken nuggets and an oily prawn omelette is considered healthy. So, regrettably, I ended up eating out the whole week.

Besides the slight problem I faced with the diet, this week was a good start to the programme. I even had excess energy after completing the training programme. So I went rollerblading a few times with my army friends. I recently picked up rollerblading because it allows me to burn calories without putting too much stress on my knees. I am now hooked on it. I like to rollerblade at night as it is less crowded and I can speed over longer distances. Rollerblading at night also allows me to enjoy the activity more privately. In the day, the park is often crowded and sometimes people stop me for autographs. I am quite happy to oblige, but it is quite dangerous for them to approach me while I am rollerblading as I may not be able to stop in time and may crash into them. Also, stopping abruptly on the track could be dangerous for cyclists and other rollerbladers.

> I eat almost anything and
> have a voracious appetite.

WEEK 2

After the honeymoon period last week, I was really looking forward to pushing myself hard at the workouts this week. I wasn't content with just making my muscles sore. I wanted to work them to extreme fatigue so that they would grow at a faster pace and I would regain my strength sooner. The strange thing about resistance training is that you need strength to gain more strength. The heavier you lift, the more strength you will gain. So the sooner I regained my strength, the sooner I would see results.

It is in my nature to always test my limits. At the gym, even when I feel that I can't lift anymore, I would still do that extra repetition. Or, alternatively, I would downgrade to lighter weights and lift until muscle fatigue.

My coach used to tell the whole national team that he was never worried that I would not train hard enough. What he was more concerned about was that I might over-train and get injured as a result. I remembered that when I was training for the World Wushu Championships back in 1995, I had an accident just three weeks prior to the competition date. During training, I accidentally cut myself with the broadsword and part of my left palm was nearly severed. I bled profusely and had to have 39 stitches. The doctor advised me to stop training for at least two weeks to allow my hand to heal. However, I could not wait. The championships were just three weeks away and I had to seize every opportunity to train. Moreover, it was my first attempt at competing in the broadsword event and I was not very confident. I went back to training the very next day. Even though I was training other parts of my body, the wound still bled whenever I exerted strength. To make things worse, I sprained my ankle while doing my final warm-up just 15 minutes before I was due to compete. I thought of giving up but my coach advised that I should give it my best shot since I was already there. I took to the arena and, strangely enough, I forgot all about the pain and ended up winning the gold medal!

This incident made me realise that it is all in the mind. Our bodies can actually endure a great deal more pain than we think. I felt so good not because I won gold but because I did not give up. This is the very same philosophy I adopt when it comes to the ten-week weight training programme. I really enjoy the way my muscles feel sore the day after a training session. The soreness is an indication that my muscles have been worked and are growing; this inspires me to train even harder. I managed to work in three gym sessions this week even though work was a little heavy.

I was also quite surprised that I actually stuck to the nutrition plan. I had never been on a diet before this, and my impression of diets was that they were torturous and that the food was generally bland and unappetising and that it meant going hungry all the time. I witnessed firsthand some of my colleagues going on

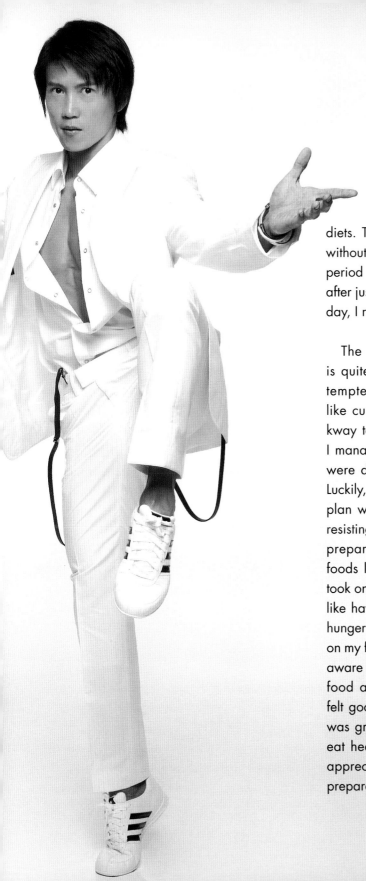

diets. There was one who lived on fish soup without rice and nothing else for an extended period of time. I tried to follow suit but gave up after just one day. Even though it was just for a day, I really felt miserable being on the diet.

The nutrition plan I'm on now, however, is quite varied. I must admit that I was still tempted to indulge in my favourite foods like curries, fried chicken, nasi lemak, beef kway teow, curry puffs and cheese fries, but I managed to stop myself, as I knew that if I were disciplined, I would see better results. Luckily, the recommended food in the nutrition plan was quite tasty, and that helped me in resisting the temptation. This week, I was more prepared too. I had stocked up on energy foods like protein shakes and muesli bars. I took one of these whenever I felt hungry or felt like having a snack. They helped to ease my hunger pangs so that I didn't feel like binging on my favourite foods. My mum was also more aware of my dietary requirements and cooked food appropriate to the diet plan. It really felt good to be able to eat at home again. I was grateful that my whole family agreed to eat healthy food with me, but most of all, I appreciated all the effort my mum put in to prepare the meals for me.

WEEK 3

The first two weeks went by smoothly and I was expecting another smooth ride this week. My strength had increased and I was looking forward to better results. The weird thing about strength and resistance training is that if you stop training you don't feel like training, but once you start training you just can't stop. Now I feel uncomfortable when my muscles don't ache.

I had initially planned to train on Monday, Wednesday and Friday. However, I was informed on Sunday night that I had filming on Monday morning. This threw my schedule off for the week. I could not postpone the training to Tuesday as it was already packed with work commitments. I desperately wanted to train, as I knew that if I missed a day this week, my efforts last week might go to waste. Worse still, I might actually run the risk of having my body regress.

On Monday evening, after a whole day of work, I managed to get to the gym at my condominium. The gym is very basic and has no free weights at all. I did my cardiovascular exercise on the treadmill and a few weight training exercises like the chest press, back row and shoulder press. Without the free weights, I could not finish the whole prescribed workout and I felt very guilty. I only felt better when I went home and did some improvised exercises that could target other parts of my body.

On Wednesday, I was called up again for filming. This time it was worse. By the time I finished work, it was nearly midnight and even my condominium's gym was closed. I had to work out, as there was no time the next day to do another session. So I went home and did the improvised exercises I covered on pages 90–97. For these exercises, the only way I could push myself was to do more repetitions instead of increasing the weight. At least, I still incorporated progressive overload into the workout. For cardiovascular exercise, I went rollerblading.

When I eventually got to the Sports Council gym on Friday, I pushed myself very hard to make up for what I missed the past few days. I tried to incorporate some of the exercises that I had to do on Monday and Wednesday into Friday's workout as well. By the end of the training session, I was really exhausted but I felt really good. All in all, I think I made the best of what was a bad situation.

When I reached home after the workout on Friday, I was greeted by a familiar smell—fish head curry. It was not just some ordinary fish head curry but that made by my grandmother. To my horror, what accompanied the curried fish head was a huge spread of goodies—chicken wrapped in pandan leaf, black pepper crab and other mouth-watering dishes. The need to immediately get at the food was overwhelming, but I managed to stop myself. Grandmother, who was in her usual jovial mood, began to urge me to try my favourite dishes. She even volunteered to serve me personally. I felt really

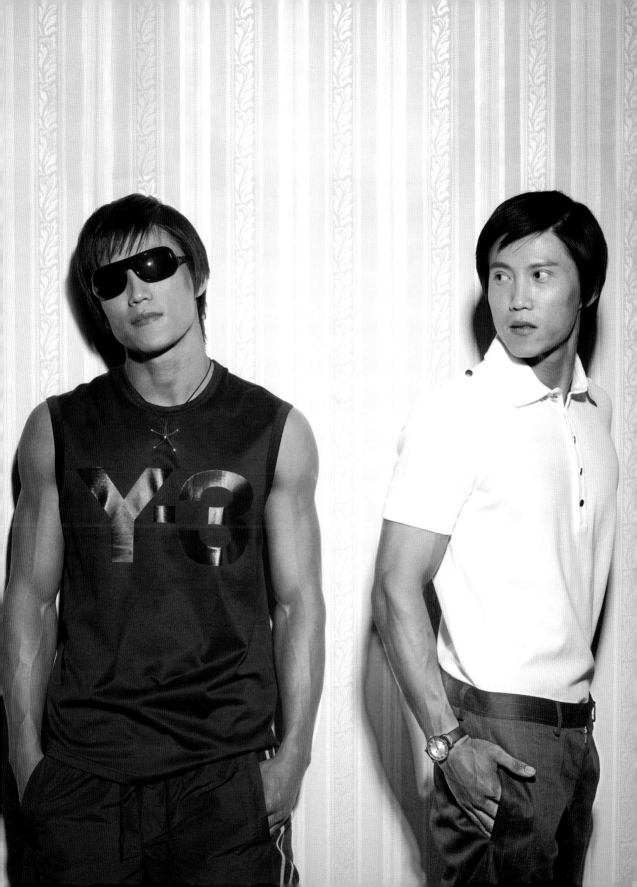

> Our bodies can actually endure a great deal more pain than we think. I felt so good not because I won gold but because I did not give up.

bad and did not know how to turn her down. I decided to tell her the truth; I thought that she would understand. How wrong could I get? She started to nag: "You are already so skinny! Still diet for what?" I had to go to my room to avoid her.

Even in my room, I found it hard not to be tempted by the food. I think I lost all appetite for muesli bars and noodle soup. They all seemed so tasteless compared to my grandmother's cooking and, at that moment, I actually hated myself for being in the programme. I only felt better when a friend agreed to accompany me for a healthy meal. Once again, my friends had come to my rescue.

WEEK 4

Last week was horrible but I managed to turn things round by improvising and not giving up. I was hoping that this week would be better—that things would fall into place and that there would be fewer disturbances. However, things never seem to go the way you want it to.

This time round, it could have been due to my over-ambitious scheduling. As usual, I planned to visit the gym on Monday, Wednesday and Friday. I knew that Monday would be a hectic day packed with filming and a rehearsal for a charity show. Yet, I thought I could squeeze in some time at the gym. Those few hours did not materialise.

We were filming a big stunt scene that day. The scene opened with me on a scrambler, chasing my on-screen love interest's kidnapper in his getaway car. The kidnapper turns the car around and knocks me off my motorcycle. I continue the chase on foot, and the kidnapper almost gets away. But I manage to 'borrow' a bicycle and eventually I catch up with the car. The sequence ends at the kidnapper's hideout where I fight him and his fellow miscreants. Although I manage to floor them, a particularly persistent kidnapper still manages to escape. To apprehend him, I have to jump on to his moving vehicle. In the end, I rescue my love interest and save the day. How else could the story end?

Because of my wushu background, producers and directors expect me to do my own stunts

because this would look better and more believable on television. For these reasons, I do nearly all the stunts in the television programmes I star in. For the filming this week, we started with the part where I had to jump on to the car first. This sequence was actually quite challenging. Although I had done this kind of stunt before, I still felt the pressure. Of utmost importance was coordination with the stunt driver of the vehicle. If the timing was off, I could fall flat on my face. In the end, I had to do the take five times from different angles with an additional N-G (no good) take or two.

Then came the really exhausting shot: I had to maintain a constant sprint behind a moving truck. The camera, the whole crew and the director were on the truck while I gave chase behind. The road, which ran mostly upslope, was uneven and winding. The sun was scorching, and to top it off, I was clad in a jacket, shirt and pants. Could I have asked for worse conditions? The shot was made all the more difficult by the fact that I had to run at the same pace as the moving vehicle; a little slower or faster than the truck and the shot would go out of focus. Each take required me to run about 200 to 300 metres and it eventually took a total of ten takes to complete the sequence. That meant that I actually sprinted for a total of two to three kilometres! My legs felt as if they were giving way on the tenth sprint, but I did not want to stop. Somehow, everybody agreed that the tenth was the best.

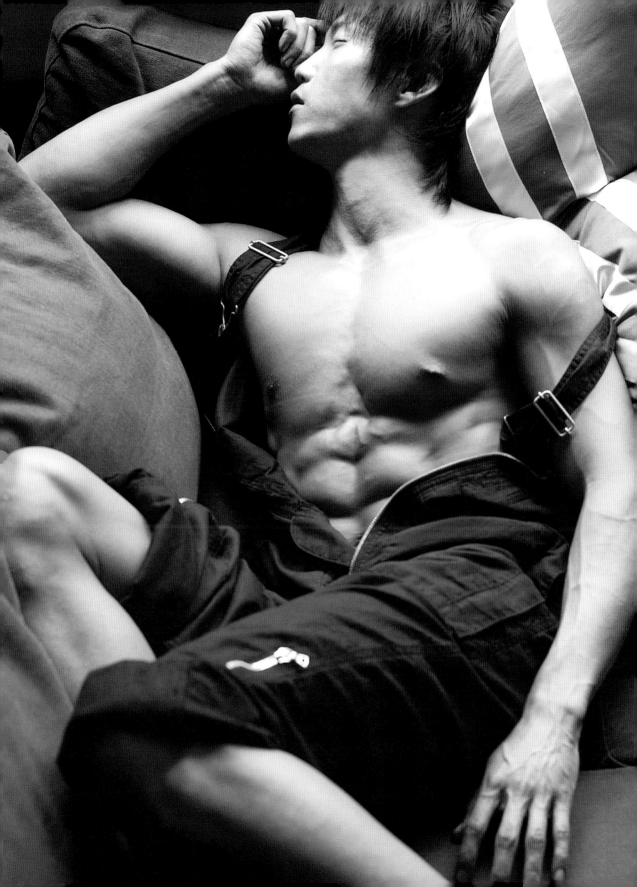

"

I do nearly all the stunts in the television programmes I star in.

"

That was still not the end. After the sprints, I had to do the scrambler sequence. By then, I was already totally sapped. Despite my fatigue, I hurriedly got into position. However, when I put on the motorcycle helmet, I started to see stars and felt short of breath. I had to ask the director for an additional 10 minutes to recover. I was grateful that he readily agreed. After the rest, the scrambler sequence was completed without a hitch.

Then came the cycling part. Initially, the cycling was relatively easy as I was on a paved road but then I had to cycle off the track on uneven grass patches. This was a classic example of progression for cardiovascular exercise—incorporating instability. I used another tonne of energy doing that sequence.

Finally, just when I thought filming was over, I was called to 'fight' with the kidnappers at the hideout. By the time we got to the fighting sequence, I was already soaked in sweat and

I had not an ounce of energy left. Luckily, we could not finish the scene; I had to be released for the charity show rehearsal. The filming for the fight scene would have to be continued some other day. I was very grateful to live to fight another day. I knew I could make the scene look better.

So, the few hours that I thought I had for the gym did not materialise. In hindsight, even if I had had those few hours, I would not have gone to the gym. I realised I wasn't superman.

By the time I reached home, I was beat. I lay slumped on the sofa and didn't want to move. The thought of working out did cross my mind, but I knew that physically I wasn't up to it anymore. I am human after all.

The rest of the week, however, didn't turn out to be as bad. I was glad that after that exhausting Monday, I managed to go for all my workouts as scheduled.

WEEK 5

I am quite proud of myself. Although my workload has been extremely heavy these past weeks, somehow I managed to squeeze in enough time for my workouts. I was also quite pleased with my self-discipline: I did not give in to my cravings. But the lure of good food got the better of me this week.

It was one of my instructors' birthday. A few of my students and instructors suggested organising a celebration, and I thought that it was a great idea. I could also use this opportunity to thank my instructors and students for their help in setting up the wushu school and its website. Yet, somehow I knew that I would be in trouble, nutrition-wise, once I decided to join in the celebration. However, on this occasion, I rationalised that it would be worthwhile to make such a sacrifice. Moreover, I have been so busy recently that I had had no time to myself. This celebration could be the perfect occasion for me to give myself a treat and recharge.

On Saturday, the whole bunch of us went bowling, rollerblading and cycling in the afternoon and we thoroughly enjoyed ourselves. I was pleasantly surprised that many of my students still had the energy for play after the comprehensive wushu lesson in the morning. But then again, who doesn't have energy to play?

In the evening, I treated everyone to Indo-Thai food. We were all hungry after a long day of play and we ordered a feast: tom yam soup, pomelo salad, chicken wrapped in pandan leaf, deep-fried fish with mango, olive rice, chicken green curry and much, much more. Initially, I had some doubts about indulging, but when the dishes were served, all caution was thrown to the wind. For once, in a very long time, I was really enjoying myself with my friends without having to think too much about anything. Call it an excuse, but it really recharged me.

After the meal, we proceeded to a cyber café for a preview of the school's website. Everyone was especially creative and contributed lots of ideas to improve wufangsingapore.com.

I was still feeling high when I got home. For once, I was not slumped on the floor, gasping for air, but punching the air and prancing around like a little kid. Then reality struck, and I realised that I had over-eaten. I didn't exactly regret my decision, but I felt a little guilty that I had let Fahma, my nutritionist, down. To redeem myself, I decided to go for a jog despite it being already 1 am.

I had only planned on a short run but it was so therapeutic that I found myself running for quite a distance. The night was so serene; the fronds of the palm trees were swaying in the wind and the sea was lapping gently onto the beach. I could not see clearly what was in front of me but all I knew was that I was taken by this overwhelming need to run. I finally realised the meaning of taking a break in order to travel a longer distance. I guessed it was well taken in the end.

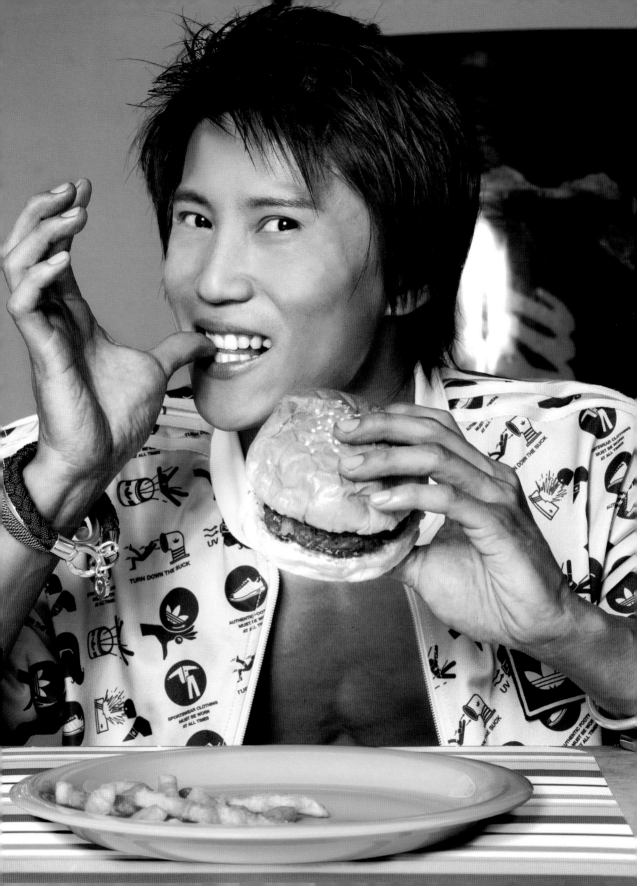

"I finally realised the meaning of taking a break in order to travel a longer distance. I guessed it was well taken in the end.

WEEK 6

I indulged on food last week and felt recharged this week, really recharged. Perhaps it was just plain guilt, or maybe the break from the diet really did reinvigorate me. Whatever it was, I was raring to go this week.

For once, the week started out quite nicely. There were also not many work commitments this week besides that for my wushu school. I welcomed the start of the week with an outing under the sun—wakeboarding! To me, the best time to wakeboard is on Monday morning. With the weekend crowd back in their offices, the seas are usually empty. The waters in the morning are also calmer. Privacy, fresh air, a smooth ride, good friends and lots of laughter—what else could one ask for?

Jimboh, my wakeboarding buddy, had a new boat, and my friends and I boarded it at Punggol Marina. I was especially excited that day as it had been quite sometime since I rode out to sea. To me, wakeboarding represents something more than a sport: it is a picnic under the sun and in the middle of the sea, and is an opportunity for me to get in touch with nature. More importantly, I could chill out with my friends.

Jimboh's 'new baby' was spacious and swanky and packed a lot of engine power. With the increased power, we were able to load the boat with more sand-filled drums to create bigger wakes for bigger jumps. I found myself in top form that morning. I landed most of the tricks I tried—a few jumps,

a few different grabs, some 180s, some heel-side and toe-side backrolls, and a couple of tantrums – and everyone was ecstatic. As I rode, I felt the thrill of the adrenaline rush and, at the same time, a deep sense of peace. On the wakeboard, it was just the sea and I: no politics, no backstabbing, no fake smiles and lip service. After I finished one run, what greeted me on the boat were friendly smiles, high-fives and the warm, delicious aroma of curry rice.

I was hungry and cold, and the curry smelled really good. I nearly forgot that I was on a diet and was about to start on the curry, when I checked myself. At that point, I hated myself for giving in last week; had I not indulged last week, I would have been able to at least have one serving of the curry. I was actually at the point of giving in to my hunger when my good friend Celia remarked that she could see improvements in my body definition. Her compliment sort of woke me up and motivated me to persevere. Suddenly, the curry didn't seem half as appetising.

I went home feeling very proud of myself for resisting the curry under those conditions. Celia's words struck me again and I started to wonder if her words were true. The narcissistic side of me took hold and I began examining my physique in the mirror. Maybe it was just the tan or maybe my body really had improved but I liked what I saw in the mirror. (I can't believe I am saying this!) Wakeboarding really does provide a good workout for the whole body, especially the shoulders, arms back, abs and butt. I realised that my good performance at sea today was due to the strength that I had gained from my training. Having seen the results of my hard work, I resolved to train even harder as I knew that I could still do even better.

Looking at myself in the mirror reminded me of what David Gan once told me. When I first started out in the entertainment industry, I didn't know a thing about grooming and making myself look good. David told me that stars have to want to look good. He made me realise that an actor can only explore and truly flesh out the many characters he or she plays when they are confident about themselves.

This on-screen confidence, in part, comes from looking good. Moreover, it is the actor's responsibility, David explained, to present his or her best side to the audience.

The rest of the week was also great. I worked harder than before at my gym sessions and even went rollerblading one night. I was so motivated that the thought of binging did not even cross my mind. Maybe the results I saw spurred me to train harder. Maybe the indulgence last week was well taken. Or maybe I had enough rest this week so I could work harder. No matter what it was, this week was the most fruitful so far in terms of my workout and diet plans.

"

When I first started out in the entertainment industry, I didn't know a thing about grooming…along the way I learnt that actors can only explore and truly flesh out the many characters they play when they are confident about themselves. This on-screen confidence, in part, comes from looking good.

"

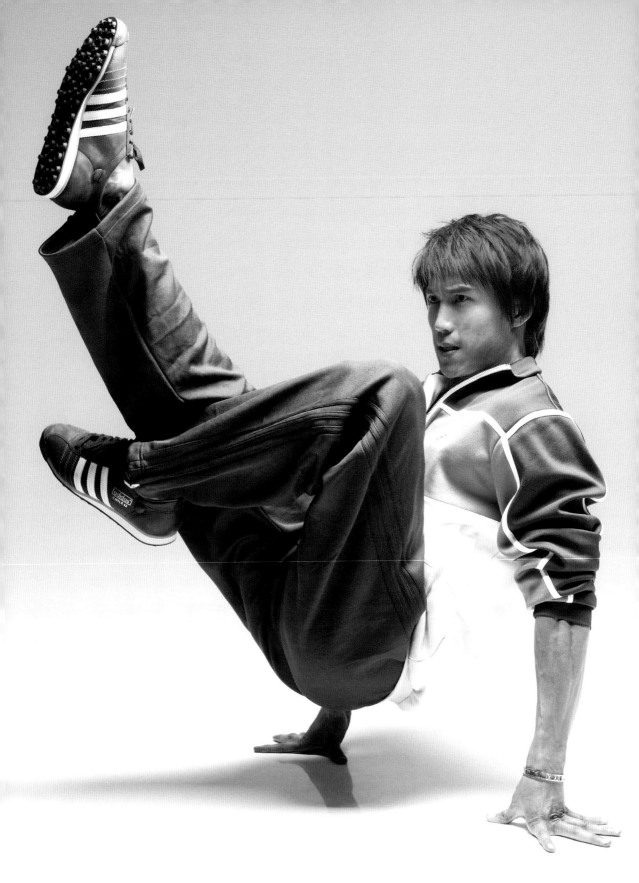

WEEK 7

There is a saying that 'the rich get richer'. So in sports the good get better. I know this because I have firsthand experience of it in my sporting career, and once again this week. The hard work of the past weeks began to yield results and these results motivated me to work even harder. Other parts of my life likewise started to show results, and I drew my inspiration from them.

This was grading week for my wushu students. Initially, I was a little apprehensive about the performance of some of the weaker students. But after the first test, I realised that my worries were unfounded. Many of these students showed tremendous improvement. I was even more pleasantly surprised that this was not limited to the weaker students but applied across the board. I found out that my students had organised extra training lessons to help one another. Their progress also came from their amazing drive: those who were in danger of failing, wanted to pass; those who passed with bronze standards, wanted silver and gold; while those who were of gold standard, wanted to be the best. These students probably had to make many personal sacrifices to achieve these results.

My students' dedication and will to succeed reminded me of the time I was training competitively. I was selected for the national wushu team at the age of 13. I had to train six times a week. The bus journey from my home in Jurong West to the Singapore National Wushu Federation in Tanjong Katong took one and a half hours and felt like eternity to me; all I wanted was to get to the Federation as fast as possible. Throughout those bus trips, I would visualise wushu moves in my mind in preparation for my lessons.

By the time I was 15, I was already representing Singapore in my first Southeast Asian (SEA) Games. Training sessions got tougher but transport was more convenient—there was the MRT. The MRT was more comfortable, and I would sometimes doze off during the journey. I participated in my second SEA Games when I was 17. By then, I was training full-time 12 times a week. I won my first gold medal that year.

I won gold at the World Wushu Championships when I was 19. This victory was especially sweet, as I had to go through hell to get it. I was assigned to the commandos unit for my national service, and I had to juggle full-time commando training with full-time wushu training. The Sports Council had applied for my release to train full-time. My unit agreed on condition that I continue military training everyday after my wushu lessons.

I ended up doing two jobs. My usual day started with physical exercises with my unit. By mid-morning, I would be released for wushu training. After an intensive workout with my coach, I would return to camp to continue training with my platoon mates. In the evening,

I would make the journey back to the wushu federation for training again. It became so taxing that the journeys between the military camp and federation soon became much-needed respites from the physical demands of both jobs.

Soon, the naps I took while commuting became my only source of rest, and this was not enough for me to recover from all that training. It was only when my last reserves of energy were sapped that I voiced my concern to the Federation. Fortunately, I was released from my unit to train for three months.

Today, I see the same determination in many of my students. Many of them stay back after classes to consult me on ways to improve. Many parents also show their support and commitment by personally ferrying their kids to and from my school. This not only encourages their children, but encourages me too. The school has come together like a family, its members helping one another, nudging everyone along. Hopefully, this family spirit would take us far. Most of the elements for success are there. What the school needs now is perseverance and time.

Persistence is also what I need to finish my workout programme. This week, it came easily. The sources of my motivation were everywhere: from the results that I had achieved so far, from the spirit to excel shown by my students and from the gratitude of my students' parents. There were a few times this week, however, when I thought about sinful foods. In fact, I even gave in to my cravings once, but I made up for it by going for a run after that. I increased the intensity of my workouts, increasing the number of sets as well as the weight I carried. I know I won't fail. How could I fail with a whole army behind me?

"
How could I fail with a
whole army behind me?
"

WEEK 8

I was working out at the gym on Monday morning when a good friend called me. When he realised that I was at the gym, he asked if he could join me as he was on leave for two weeks and had nothing much to do. I agreed without hesitation; this friend of mine had been wanting to try out resistance training for quite a while. Having a workout buddy can also be a very good way of motivating yourself. For me, the sight of a friend trying his best spurs me to want to give my best too.

I received permission from the Sports Council to admit my friend to the gym. During the workout, I took on the role of trainer, correcting my friend's posture and encouraging him to complete his repetitions. My friend also helped me with the weights when I needed a little assistance finishing my last repetitions. Yet, as I was helping him, I sensed that my friend was not really pushing himself.

At lunch, my friend confessed that he felt intimidated by the national athletes at the gym. He felt that they had better bodies and could lift heavier weights. Much to my surprise, he was very concerned with what they thought of him. I felt rather guilty for not being able to empathise with my friend, as I had never felt that way before when it came to anything physical. I advised my friend to concentrate on what he was doing and not think about what others thought of him. I also recounted an incident that happened during my competition days.

When I was representing Singapore in international competitions in the 1990s, I had the help of sports psychologists. The sports psychologists taught me many different techniques to cope with the mental challenges of competing: how to focus on the task at hand, how to motivate myself, how to push myself to realise my fullest potential, and how not to be psychologically affected by my opponents. One of the ways not to be intimidated by your opponents is to avoid eye contact with them or even to look at them. Different athletes have their own way to help them stay focused: some like to listen to motivational music, some like to talk to themselves, some pray, while others like to visualise their routines. For me, I prefer to be left alone to go through my routine mentally. Sometimes, I talk to myself.

I managed to apply what I had learnt at the 1997 SEA Games. At that point, I was at my physical peak. While I was warming up just before the competition, I realised that my closest competitor was stealing glances at me. We were both aware of the other's physical prowess, as we had trained together at the Beijing Shichahai Sports School. I had always performed better during training: I could jump higher, I could run faster and farther and I could lift heavier weights. That day, I could sense that he was intimidated by me as he kept looking in my direction. I knew that I had already won half the battle as I had the mental edge, but I wanted to intimidate him further.

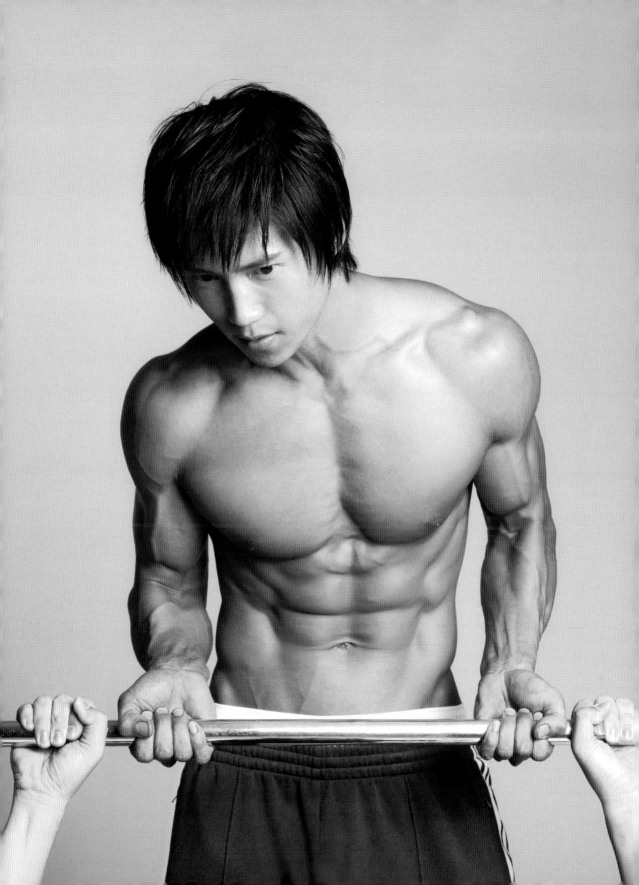

> Having a workout buddy can also be a very good way of motivating yourself. For me, the sight of a friend trying his best spurs me to want to give my best too.

I knew that my forte was my jumps, and I started to perform them in front of him. True enough, he fell into my trap.

I focused on the task at hand and managed to perform up to expectations. He, on the other hand, felt insecure, and started to over-compensate for his insecurity. In the end, his performance was full of errors, and I won the gold medal.

After hearing my story, my friend realised that he had allowed his inferiority complex to get the better of him. The next time we went to the gym, my friend was better: he did not look at the other athletes as much; he just went about doing his own workout, and was not embarrassed about the weights he carried. By the third session, he was much more comfortable and I could sense that he was pushing himself harder. It could have been because he was more familiar with the people and the environment, or maybe because what I said really did have some effect. Whatever the case, I got myself a good workout buddy.

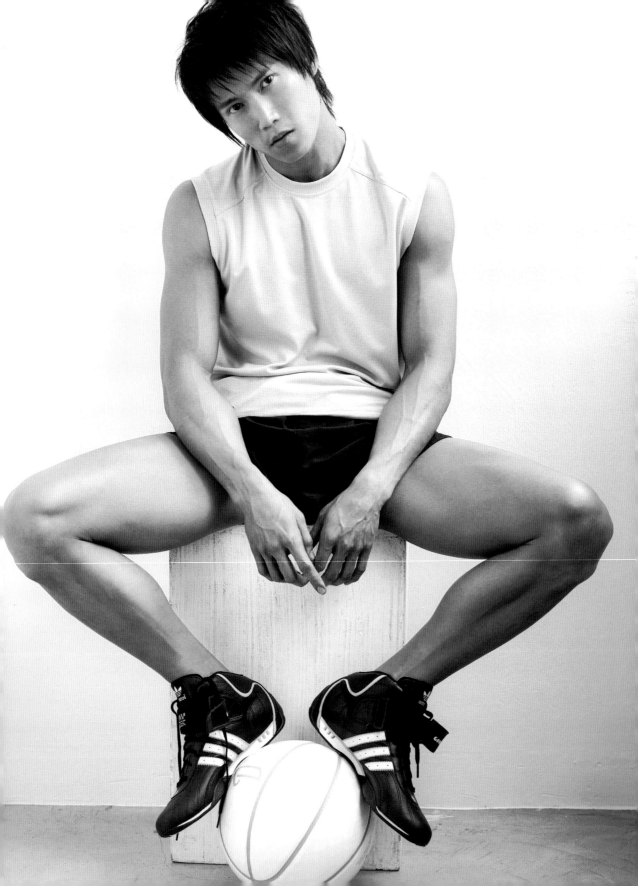

WEEK 9

It is just two weeks to the end of the programme. Up till now, I had been quite disciplined. Although I faltered a couple of times when it came to my diet, I kept religiously to the training programme. Sometimes, I even did more than what was required.

This week, my friend trained with me again. With him around, I could work even harder—when I pushed myself to the point where my muscles gave way, it was my friend who gave me a little help to finish up the repetitions. I also found it very much easier to stick to my diet with my friend joining me. In fact, my friend was more conscientious than me in this regard, and he constantly reminded me not to waver. On my part, I also encouraged him while he trained.

However, in spite of the better workouts, I somehow felt that my body was not improving fast enough. I wasn't satisfied with what I saw in the mirror. Although my muscles felt tight, they were not aching as much as when I first started the exercise regime. I missed the pain; I wanted my muscles to ache, to grow bigger. I feared that if I did not train hard enough, I would start to shrink.

But I knew that this was all psychological. What was dangerous for me was to give in to these thoughts. If I were to lift heavier weights and train any harder, my body would become too big and bulky for my liking. This was a trap I had once fallen into.

A few years ago, I was asked by the producers of Heartlanders to bulk up, as they wanted to include more scenes that featured me topless. I headed for the gym two months before filming started, and began working out. After one and a half months of training, I thought that my body was not improving. One day, I would feel that my chest was not big enough (because my arms and back were bigger) and I would intensify my chest exercises. Another day, I would think that my back was not developed enough (when in actual fact it only looked smaller because my chest had grown) and I would begin targeting my back. Soon after, I began to think that my biceps and triceps were too small. It soon became a vicious cycle. I even started taking protein shakes. Eventually, my body bulked up a lot. However, I still was not satisfied, and I continued training with ever-increasing intensity. Till one day…

I had just finished my workout at the MediaCorp gym when I ran into Zoe Tay.

"Qing Hai, please don't train anymore!" she exclaimed. "You are growing too big. Not nice anymore."

At first, I didn't believe her. I explained to her that I probably looked bigger because I had just finished a workout. Later, when I was alone in the toilet, her words started to haunt me, and I examined myself in the mirror. It was as if a veil had suddenly been lifted from my eyes.

"It was as if a veil had suddenly been lifted from my eyes. My chest was bulging. The veins in my arms and neck were so swollen they looked as if they were ready to burst."

My chest was bulging. The veins in my arms and neck were so swollen they looked as if they were ready to burst. I looked exactly like a mannequin in a Chinese physician's office. It was then that I realised that Zoe was right. I really had grown too bulky. In fact, I thought I looked like a smaller version of the Incredible Hulk and I became very alarmed, as I prefer to be lean and defined, instead of bulky and stout. After this incident, I reduced my visits to the gym and did more exercises like jogging, cycling, rollerblading, basketball, wushu and other sports to cut down on my bulk.

I wasn't going to make the same mistake. This week would be the last time I would be increasing the weights. From next week, I would train using the same weights, only increasing the repetitions. I would also spend more time doing other forms of exercises, such as stretching, wushu, wakeboarding, rollerblading, cycling, basketball and jogging. Stretching also helps as it not only warms up the muscles and prevents injury, but also makes them more flexible and looking longer and more beautiful. Wushu is very good for overall conditioning and building up the smaller muscle groups. Wakeboarding lets me enjoy the sea while building up my upper body. Cycling builds up the back and lower body. Rollerblading and jogging help me de-stress and, at the same time, burn calories. Doing a variety of exercises that work every muscle group ensures that I never turn into the Incredible Hulk again.

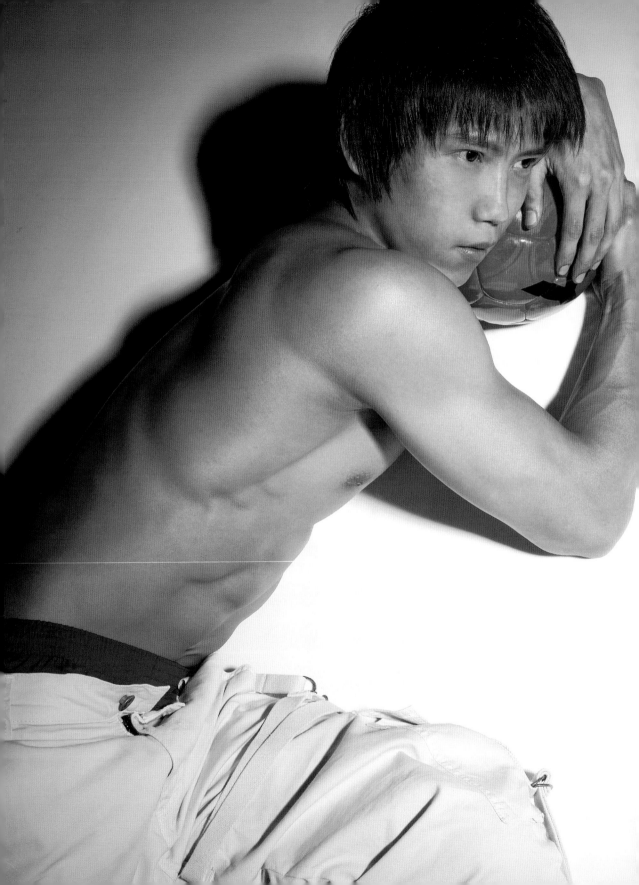

WEEK 10

The last week of the programme finally arrived. My gym buddy had to return to work, and I was alone again. My work schedule had gotten tighter too. But I was motivated to complete the programme. Following the nutrition plan this week was not difficult; I had already followed it for nine weeks, so what was one more week? I also worked harder at the gym to make sure that I met my targets.

As I finished the last set of exercises, and as I lay down on my rooftop garden for a suntan, I felt lighter, as if a huge weight had been lifted off my back. But then it occurred to me that meeting my targets had become secondary. So what if I missed my target by 1 per cent? I wasn't going to kill myself over this little 'failure'. What was more important was the process: the process of pushing myself to the limit, of resisting temptation, of knowing my body better and of self-discovery.

Despite the ups and downs, I am proud of what I had learnt and achieved in these ten weeks. Now, I know that I can say no to my favourite foods, that taking a break is not always bad and that I would eventually succeed if I take on all challenges, one small step at a time. I realised that these ten weeks were a microcosm of my life: the ups, the downs, the rebounds and the constant persevering.

My career in the entertainment industry began when I became a finalist in Star Search 1997. The first few years were quite good,

but then suddenly I fell into a rut. I could not derive any satisfaction from my job. I lost my way, and there were times when I wondered if I was really suitable for the industry. Maybe I was too brash, maybe I was too impatient, maybe I wasn't flexible enough, or maybe I just wasn't good enough.

I think I am really blessed in spite of all these failings. Since young, I have had the great fortune of meeting people who, in times of need, have lent me a helping hand. This time round, my benefactors were my friends and family. Some encouraged me, some helped me put things into perspective, and some showed me the light. Suddenly, things didn't look half as bad.

I started to take pleasure in the little things in life. Strangers walking up to me to say that I have improved and that they enjoy watching me act. The friends from my fan club, who constantly remind me of their support at media events and through correspondence. The instructors and students (and their parents) of my wushu school who took the time to celebrate my birthday by ambushing me with water bombs. Television directors and other friends from the entertainment industry enlightening me on the future of our industry and my future in the industry. Old friends calling me to say 'hi'. My parents and family, who have always been there for me.

I realised that many people were behind me, wanting to see me go on, wanting to see me succeed. I told myself that I couldn't give up; if I did I would be letting all of them down. I always thought that it was wushu training that has given me the capacity to endure hardship, a never-say-die attitude and a will to succeed. This was what I believed until a mentor told me otherwise. He said that I had all these qualities already in me and that was why I could become a wushu world champion. Suddenly, my perspective on the world changed. I knew that I had it in me to endure, to fight, and to excel. I proved this to myself in these ten weeks and I know that I can also do it in life.

As I lay on the rooftop, the sky looked bright and sunny. It was so bright that I had to squint to look up at the sky. A flock of birds flew over me and into the distance. Things never felt so great. All I wanted to do was to bask in this little moment of self-appreciation. It occurred to me that I would be stepping on to the measuring scale tomorrow. But I think I didn't care if I had succeeded or not. Or did I?

"

I realised that many
people were behind
me, wanting to see me
go on, wanting to see
me succeed.

"

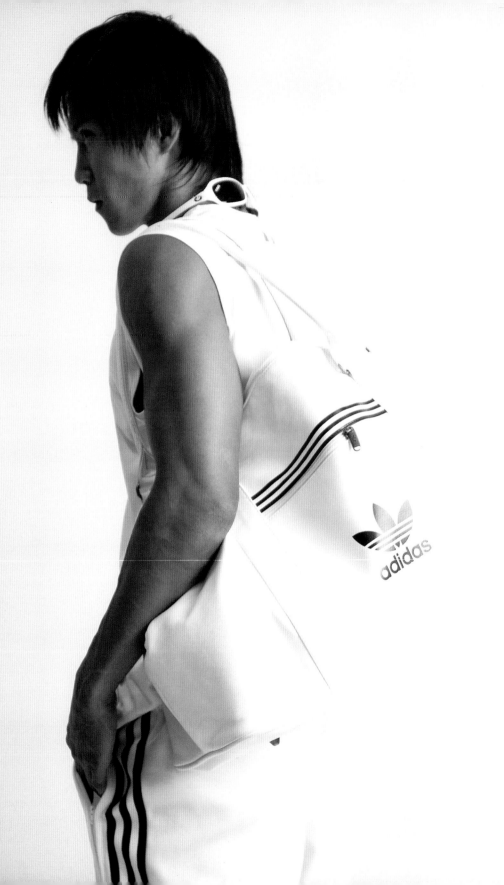

Week eleven and after— maintenance

Finally, the ten weeks are over. Have I achieved my goals? After stepping on the scales, these are my results:

Body weight: 65 kg
Body fat percentage: 7.2%

Compared to the goals I set, I think I have done very well. Although my present body fat percentage is slightly higher than my target of 7 per cent, I did gain 1.5 kilograms of lean body mass. If I continue to work at the body fat, I know I will reach my goal in another few days or maybe a week.

Many of you, however, would have probably attained your goals. So what is next?

For me, I am going to give myself a big treat; I am going to have my favourite fried chicken, my grandmother's curry chicken and ice cream. I am also going to take a break from the gym for a week.

Although I'll be taking a break from the gym, I know I will soon be back there again with a vengeance. I have finally regained the fitness that I lost and I am not going to give it up easily. I'm sure those of you who have hit your targets will be equally reluctant to give up your hard-earned fitness.

Maintaining your fitness, lean body mass and body fat composition requires the same discipline and hard work that we have put in over the last ten weeks. For this maintenance phase, we have to start setting goals again. This time round,

I will probably set more modest goals: I want to lose a further 1.2 per cent of body fat and I wish to maintain the same amount of lean muscle mass. The whole cycle repeats itself, but this time round with new dynamics because my goals are different. If you are still not happy with how you look, then set yourself more aggressive goals. Remember this: you have to continually set yourself new goals or you run the risk of not being motivated enough to continue your training. By not doing anything, everything you have achieved so far will go to waste.

Fitness programme

By now, my body should be accustomed to the exercises I have been doing for the past ten weeks. To get more results, I will need to change things a little—I will have to incorporate more progressive overload.

As my goals for the maintenance phase are quite modest and I am not looking at putting on additional muscle mass, I will not need to increase the weights that I lift during my strength and resistance workouts. Instead, I will perform more sets and repetitions, alter the angles of the exercises and reduce the speed at which I perform individual repetitions. Alternatively, I could circuit train; this entails performing one set of each exercise in succession with very little rest in between. However, whatever I do, I will still have to push myself to the limit, to the point of muscle failure.

I will also have to increase the intensity of my cardiovascular exercises. I will adjust the ratio of my cardiovascular exercises to strength and resistance training from 25:75 to 30:70. The same rules of progression apply to the cardiovascular exercises. Maintaining the same level of intensity is not going to be effective.

Nutrition plan for the next ten weeks

I have set myself the goal of losing 1.2 per cent, or 780 grams, of body fat in the next ten weeks. This means that I have to lose a total of 6,006 calories. With my new weight, my daily caloric intake can be calculated in this way:

My new BMR is 1624.2
My new daily metabolism is 2598.7
Calories I need to lose each day is 85.8
Calories I can consume each day is 2512.9

With my new weight and goal, I can probably consume 2,500 calories each day. Once in a while, I will be able to give myself a treat, but I will have to compensate by training a little harder.

Eating right on all occasions

To master the art of maintenance, we have to master the art of anticipation. We might as well throw our workout and nutrition plans out the window if we do not plan for the times when we may be faced with the temptation to overeat.

> Maintaining your fitness, lean body mass and body fat composition requires the same discipline and hard work that we have put in over the last ten weeks.

I do let myself go once in a while, even as often as once a week. But what happens to the other days of the week? How do we work around social dinners, family outings and the many other occasions that often lead us to consume more calories than we require? The answer is to anticipate and prepare.

1. At work and at home

At my workplace, colleagues often bring food such as curry puffs, cakes and chicken rice to the film set. These foods can be very fattening and unhealthy. I often tell myself that I will not touch these snacks. But then, when it comes to the crunch (especially when I am bored between takes), I often make excuses. I will convince myself that having just that one curry puff or slice of cake will not do much damage to my diet. This, however, is a very bad move. That one piece very often leads to another, and before you know it, your nutrition plan is dashed.

My grandmother often comes over to my place to cook her sumptuous curries and her trademark dishes such as bubur chacha, black pepper crab, assam fish head and chicken wrapped in pandan leaf. I know that I cannot, ordinarily, ever resist my grandmother's cooking. So I think I am going to let myself go when it comes to my grandmother's food. However, in order to indulge in my grandmother's cooking, I cannot succumb to the other food temptations that I encounter.

One way of dealing with these temptations is to make sure that I never go hungry. I can do so by making sure that I always have some fruit in my bag. Whenever I feel like eating or munching, I will eat the fruit. This also means that I can keep track of the number of calories I am consuming.

Although I have no children of my own, I often observe that some of my friends eat what their children leave behind during mealtimes, perhaps to avoid wasting food. As children's food is very high in calories, you may end up overeating and harming your own health.

2. Business functions, wedding dinners and formal occasions

I often have to attend many functions in my line of work. These business functions vary from appreciation dinners, wrap parties after a certain show ends, celebratory dinners for a show's good ratings and many others. Many times, the food that is served in these functions is deep-fried and high in calories and cholesterol. Before attending these functions, I make sure I take an afternoon snack of fruit, yoghurt or an energy bar, so that I do not get there feeling hungry and start overeating. If possible, I will take my dinner first before going to these functions. When I am not hungry, the temptation to eat will be greatly diminished.

Many social occasions involve indulging in alcohol. Although I am not a big fan of alcohol, I do not mind an occasional wine or beer. Wine contains 25 calories an ounce, beer 60 calories an ounce and hard liquor 100 calories an ounce. These calories do not trigger satiation mechanisms in the body. This means that although we are consuming

That one piece very often leads to another, and before you know it, your nutrition plan is dashed.

calories when we drink alcohol, our bodies are not responding to them, and our hunger is unabated. On a side note, one olive is 40 calories and high in fat. So if your drink comes with an olive, it is another 40 calories. You might want to give the olive a miss.

I will try to adjust my daily nutrition plan if I know that I am going drinking. I try to limit my intake to two glasses, which is about 4 ounces. That means that for that particular day, I will have to eat less.

3. Buffets

Everybody knows that the buffet table is filled with the biggest calorie bombs. How do I navigate this minefield? I fill up my plate with fruit, salad with vinaigrette, sliced turkey or chicken, and made to order vegetable omelettes. Of course, I will still have a smidgeon of my favourite dishes, but after loading up with the healthier food, I will have very little space for the sinful stuff.

4. Flights

Standard airline food is a sodium, calorie and cholesterol nightmare. You can avoid airline meals by ordering a special meal for yourself in advance. Order a fruit platter, salad with vinaigrette (other dressings such as thousand island, even low-fat versions, can be very high in calories), or even cold soba noodles. Alternatively, you can pack your own food and ask the flight attendant to have it heated up.

"
Do not sacrifice technique and form for a heavier weight.
"

Session 1	Week:			Week:			Week:		
	Reps	Sets	Weight used	Reps	Sets	Weight used	Reps	Sets	Weight used
Dumbbell bench press									
Squats									
Chin ups									
Dynamic dumbbell lunges									
Standing dumbbell bicep curls									
Reverse flyes									
Standing woodchopper									
Back extensions									
Session 2									
Incline bench press									
Leg press									
Seated dumbbell shoulder press									
Seated row									
Dumbbell flyes									
Calf raises									
Tricep pushdowns									
Alternate arm and leg extensions									
Session 3									
Bench press									
Squats									
Lat pulldowns									
45 degree dumbbell lunges									
Barbell upright row									
Standing reverse woodchopper									
Back extensions									

Exercises to be done at every session: Toe touches, Back extensions side bend, Lower abs, Gymnastic sit-ups and Static hold.

" ... my perspective on the world changed. I knew that I had it in me to endure, to fight, and to excel. I proved this to myself in these ten weeks and I know that I can also do it in life. "

Bibliography

Karas, Jim. *Business plan for the body.* Three Rivers Press: New York, 2001.
Peterson, Gunnar. *G-Force.* HarperCollins: New York, 2005.
Weider, Ben and Joe Weider with Danjiel Gastelu. *The edge.* Avery: New York, 2003.

Acknowledgements

Many thanks to Ivy Low and Mei Ho of the Artiste Management Division, MediaCorp Studios for co-managing this project.

Fitness Consultants
James Wong, Singapore Sports Council
Nelson Chong, California Fitness Singapore

Nutrition Consultant
Fahma Sunarja, Singapore Sports Council

Photography
Lifestyle photos by E Henry
Exercise photos by Elements By the Box

Styling and Hair
David Gan, Passion Hair Salon

Styling Assistant
Joshua Chung

Grooming
Ros Chan, Passion Hair Salon

Clothes, Accessories and Fitness Equipment
adidas/adidas Originals
Hugo Boss
NewUrbanMale.com
Y3 by BlackJack
Tiffany and Co.
Fitness First

All exercise photos were taken on location at California Fitness Singapore, Bugis.